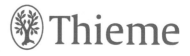

Microsurgical Basics and Bypass Techniques

Evgenii Belykh, MD, PhD
Neurosurgery Research Fellow
Department of Neurosurgery
Barrow Neurological Institute
Phoenix, Arizona
Assistant Professor
Department of Neurosurgery
Irkutsk State Medical University
Irkutsk, Russia

Nikolay L. Martirosyan, MD, PhD
Neurosurgery Fellow
Department of Neurosurgery
University of Arizona
Tucson, Arizona

M. Yashar S. Kalani, MD, PhD
Vice Chair and Associate Professor
Director of Skull Base and Neurovascular Surgery
Departments of Neurosurgery and Neuroscience
University of Virginia School of Medicine
Charlottesville, Virginia

Peter Nakaji, MD
Professor and Horace W. Steele Chair in Neurosurgical Innovation and Education
Program Director, Neurosurgery Residency Program
Department of Neurosurgery
Barrow Neurological Institute
Phoenix, Arizona

Series Editors
Peter Nakaji, MD
Vadim A. Byvaltsey, MD, PhD
Robert F. Spetzler, MD

Thieme
New York • Stuttgart • Delhi • Rio de Janeiro

Library of Congress Cataloging-in-Publication Data

Names: Belykh, Evgenii G., author. | Martirosyan, Nikolay L., author. | Kalani, Yashar, author. | Nakaji, Peter, author.

Title: Microsurgical basics and bypass techniques / Evgenii G. Belykh, Nikolay L. Martirosyan, M.Yashar S. Kalani, Peter Nakaji.

Description: New York : Thieme, [2020] | Includes bibliographical references and index. | Summary: "All neurosurgeons must undergo rigorous training in the laboratory and practice bypass techniques repetitively before performing microneurosurgery on a patient. Microsurgical Basics and Bypass Techniques by Evgenii Belykh, Nikolay Martirosyan, and M. Yashar S. Kalani is a comprehensive yet succinct manual on fundamental laboratory techniques rarely included in clinical textbooks. The resource simplifies repetitive microsurgical practice in the laboratory by providing a menu of diverse, progressively challenging exercises. Step-by-step instructions accompanied by easy-to-understand illustrations, expert commentary, and videos effectively bridge the gap between laboratory practice and operating room performance. The book starts with an opening chapter on four founding principles of microsurgical practice inherited from great thinkers and concludes with a chapter featuring cerebrovascular bypass cases. Chapters 2-8 offer a complete one-week curriculum, with a different lab exercise each day, focused on learning basic microsurgery skills"– Provided by publisher.

Identifiers: LCCN 2019027137 | ISBN 9781626235304 (softcover) | ISBN 9781626235311 (ebook)

Subjects: MESH: Microsurgery–methods Classification: LCC RD33.6 | NLM WO 512 | DDC 617.059–dc23

LC record available at https://lccn.loc.gov/2019027137

© 2020 Thieme Medical Publishers, Inc.

Thieme Publishers New York
333 Seventh Avenue, New York, NY 10001 USA
+1 800 782 3488, customerservice@thieme.com

Thieme Publishers Stuttgart
Rüdigerstrasse 14, 70469 Stuttgart, Germany
+49 [0]711 8931 421, customerservice@thieme.de

Thieme Publishers Delhi
A-12, Second Floor, Sector-2, Noida-201301
Uttar Pradesh, India
+91 120 45 566 00, customerservice@thieme.in

Thieme Publishers Rio de Janeiro, Thieme Publicações Ltda.
Edifício Rodolpho de Paoli, 25º andar
Av. Nilo Peçanha, 50 – Sala 2508,
Rio de Janeiro 20020-906 Brasil
+55 21 3172-2297 / +55 21 3172-1896
www.thiemerevinter.com.br

Barrow Neurological Institute holds the copyright to all diagnostic images, photographs, intraoperative videos, animations, and art, including the cover art, used in this work and the accompanying digital content, unless otherwise stated. Used with permission from Barrow Neurological Institute, Phoenix, Arizona.

Cover design: Thieme Publishing Group
Typesetting by Thomson Digital, Noida, India
Cover art: Peter M. Lawrence, MS

Printed in The United States of America
by King Printing Co., Inc.   5 4 3 2 1

ISBN 978-1-62623-530-4

Also available as an e-book:
eISBN 978-1-62623-531-1

Important note: Medicine is an ever-changing science undergoing continual development. Research and clinical experience are continually expanding our knowledge, in particular our knowledge of proper treatment and drug therapy. Insofar as this book mentions any dosage or application, readers may rest assured that the authors, editors, and publishers have made every effort to ensure that such references are in accordance with **the state of knowledge at the time of production of the book.**

Nevertheless, this does not involve, imply, or express any guarantee or responsibility on the part of the publishers in respect to any dosage instructions and forms of applications stated in the book. **Every user is requested to examine carefully** the manufacturers' leaflets accompanying each drug and to check, if necessary in consultation with a physician or specialist, whether the dosage schedules mentioned therein or the contraindications stated by the manufacturers differ from the statements made in the present book. Such examination is particularly important with drugs that are either rarely used or have been newly released on the market. Every dosage schedule or every form of application used is entirely at the user's own risk and responsibility. The authors and publishers request every user to report to the publishers any discrepancies or inaccuracies noticed. If errors in this work are found after publication, errata will be posted at www.thieme.com on the product description page.

Some of the product names, patents, and registered designs referred to in this book are in fact registered trademarks or proprietary names even though specific reference to this fact is not always made in the text. Therefore, the appearance of a name without designation as proprietary is not to be construed as a representation by the publisher that it is in the public domain.

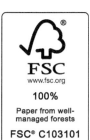

To my wife Liudmila, for wholeheartedly supporting me in my journey. To my mother Olga and to the memory of my father Georgiy, who taught me by their example the importance of sacrifice, kindness, passion for care, and striving for excellence. I am indebted to my teachers Mark C. Preul, Peter Nakaji, and Vadim A. Byvaltsev for infusing me with their spirit of curiosity and for being constant sources of wisdom and inspiration.

Evgenii Belykh, MD

Dedicated to my family, for their love and endless support.

Nikolay L. Martirosyan, MD

To Joseph M. Zabramski, who took a young intern's request seriously and spent endless hours teaching me the basics of bypass surgery. To Robert F. Spetzler, whose dedication to excellence at work and balance in life is an inspiration. To Cameron G. McDougall, who through outstanding surgical acumen and thoughtfulness in case selection taught me much about cerebrovascular disease. Thank you all for all your support and friendship over the years.

M. Yashar S. Kalani, MD, PhD

To all who, like me, are constantly learning, and to all who give back by teaching: my colleagues, my residents, my students, and especially my family.

Peter Nakaji, MD

Contents

Video Contents ix

Foreword x

Preface xi

Acknowledgments xiv

Contributors xv

1 The Philosophy of Microsurgical Practice: Four Founding Principles Inherited from
   the Great Thinkers 1
   Evgenii Belykh and Peter Nakaji

2 Day 1: The Organization of the Microsurgical Laboratory: Necessary Tools and
   Equipment 4
   Evgenii Belykh, Nikolay L. Martirosyan, and Mark C. Preul

3 Day 2: Dry-Laboratory Microsurgical Training: Techniques and Manual Skills 26
   Evgenii Belykh and Nikolay L. Martirosyan

4 Day 3: Wet-Laboratory Microsurgical Training: Basic Principles for Working with
   Laboratory Animals 56
   Evgenii Belykh and Nikolay L. Martirosyan

5 Day 4: Exercise Set 1: Basic Arterial Anastomoses 65
   Evgenii Belykh and Nikolay L. Martirosyan

6 Day 5: Exercise Set 2: Deep Field Anastomoses and Complex Vascular
   Reconstructions 75
   Evgenii Belykh and Nicolay L. Martirosyan

7 Day 6: Exercises: Kidney Autotransplantation, Supermicrosurgery, and
   Aneurysm Clipping 81
   Evgenii Belykh and Nikolay L. Martirosyan

8 Day 7: Models for Microneurosurgical Training and Schedules for Training 87
   Evgenii Belykh, Vadim A. Byvaltsev, Mark C. Preul, Peter Nakaji

9 Possible Bypass Errors 94
   Evgenii Belykh and Peter Nakaji

10 Translation of Laboratory Skills: Indications for Bypass in Neurosurgery 99
    Evgenii Belykh, M. Yashar S. Kalani, Vadim A. Byvaltsev, and Peter Nakaji

11 Case Examples of Cerebrovascular Bypass 118
    M. Yashar S. Kalani, Ken-ichiro Kikuta, and Evgenii Belykh

12 Postscript 127

Index 129

Video Contents

Video 3.1 The reverse holding technique of holding short microforceps.

Video 3.2 The index push technique of holding short microforceps.

Video 3.3 The traditional technique of holding short microforceps.

Video 3.4 Techniques of holding short straight microscissors.

Video 3.5 The reverse holding technique of holding short straight microscissors.

Video 3.6 The index push technique of holding short straight microscissors.

Video 3.7 The traditional technique of holding short straight microscissors.

Video 3.8 The traditional technique of holding long bayonet microscissors.

Video 3.9 The reverse holding technique (also known as Japanese style) of holding long bayonet microscissors.

Video 3.10 The index push technique of holding long bayonet microscissors.

Video 3.11 The chopsticks technique of holding long bayonet microscissors.

Video 3.12 Technique of picking up a needle from a flat surface.

Video 3.13 Knot-tying method 1: intermittent suture grasping.

Video 3.14 Knot-tying method 2: constant hold of one suture.

Video 3.15 Knot-tying method 3: constant hold of one suture and tightening in single direction.

Video 3.16 Exercise 4: untying a knot.

Video 3.17 Exercise 5: pushing the suture end.

Video 5.1 End-to-end anastomosis on the carotid artery with interrupted suture.

Video 5.2 End-to-side anastomosis on the carotid arteries with continuous suture.

Video 5.3 End-to-side anastomosis for creation of carotid–jugular arteriovenous fistula with interrupted suture.

Video 5.4 Side-to-side anastomosis for creation of femoral arteriovenous fistula with interrupted suture.

Video 6.1 Dissection of the aorta from the vena cava in a deep operative field.

Video 6.2 Suturing the venous interposition graft from the jugular vein into the carotid artery.

Video 7.1 Demonstration of kidney transplantation exercise.

Video 9.1 Demonstration of the high degree of tremor that can be caused by excessive muscle fatigue and tremor reduction with proper hand positioning.

Video 9.2 Errors in suture placement: loose suture placement, suture that displaces the adventitia inside the lumen, and overly tight suture that grabs too much of the vessel wall.

Foreword

This thoughtful compilation of basic microsurgical techniques and exercises to hone one's skills is a welcome practical addition for trainees and young neurosurgeons. Although there is never an age at which practice is not beneficial, it is when one is starting out that it is most important to make sure that basic skills are at their peak. I strongly believe that we have an obligation to our patients to be the best surgeons that we can be and, considering how the endless hours spent in the laboratory practicing bypass techniques have resulted in better patency and faster anastomoses in the operating room, this can only be attained through repetitive microsurgical practice in the laboratory. This volume simplifies this effort by providing a menu of different and progressively challenging exercises that you can practice to be at your best. I recommend this volume with enthusiasm.

Robert F. Spetzler, MD

Preface

Microsurgery has become an ingrained part of highly specialized surgical fields and even of general surgery. Modern reconstructive surgery simply could not exist without many of the elements of microsurgery. In the specialized areas of neurosurgery, microsurgery, and cardiac surgery, in particular, the main surgical steps are conducted only under optical magnification. Microsurgical skills are also quite useful in experimental surgery, because the most frequent models among experimental animals, for ethical and financial reasons, are mice and rats.

The first systematic experimentation with anastomosis on small vessels was reported by John Benjamin Murphy in 1897.[1] But only in the early 1900s did the medical world begin to recognize the importance of the vascular surgery techniques, first developed in 1902 by the French surgeon Alexis Carrel at the Rockefeller Institute for Medical Research (now Rockefeller University) in New York City; these techniques are now used primarily in the service of organ transplantation.[2] Carrel developed a method of vessel triangulation for anastomosis that used three supportive sutures. He was subsequently awarded the Nobel Prize in physiology or medicine in 1912 "in recognition of his work on vascular suture and the transplantation of blood vessels and organs." Carrel developed the foundational principles of vascular surgery (i.e., tensionless anastomosis and continuous endothelial–endothelial contact), which are still followed today—more than 100 years after he first espoused them.

The history of the development of microsurgical techniques in neurosurgery is directly connected with the invention of the operative microscope. In 1953, the German manufacturer Carl Zeiss developed and commercialized the first universal operative microscope (OPMI 1). The operative microscope was initially used quite successfully by otorhinolaryngologists and ophthalmologists, but it was adopted more slowly by other specialties. By 1957, after neurosurgeon Theodore Kurze observed otorhinolaryngology operations that used the OPMI 1, he started to train with it in the laboratory in an attempt to improve the approach to the cerebellopontine angle.[3] Whether he was interested in using it in microvascular surgery is unknown.

In the late 1950s, Julius H. Jacobson II,[4] a professor of surgery at the University of Vermont, was performing a scientific project with pharmacologists when he encountered difficulties completing an "end-to-end" anastomosis of a canine carotid artery (mean diameter: 3 mm) using Carrel's methods. Jacobson and his resident, Ernesto L. Suarez, decided to try applying microscopic magnification to their work using an OPMI 1 microscope that they found in the laboratory. The resulting images were no doubt as exciting as the first telescopic images of the moon.[5] This step forward eliminated the most substantial barrier to the development of successful microvascular surgery—the inability of the human eye to see microscopic details of the anatomy within the surgical field. In 1960, Jacobson and Suarez published their work *Microsurgery in Anastomosis of Small Vessels*.[4] Another pioneer of microvascular procedures in neurosurgery was Raymond M. P. Donaghy, who worked with Jacobson at the University of Vermont, where he established a microsurgery research and training laboratory in 1958.[6]

The possibility of microsurgical intervention in neurosurgery had been suggested previously. For example, in 1951, neurologist Charles Miller Fisher[7] had proposed the theoretical rationale for performing direct anastomoses between the branches of the external carotid artery and the internal carotid artery to bypass the occluded portion of the artery and thereby prevent ischemia. However, such an operation was technically impossible before the adoption of the microscope.

The case of a patient treated in the Zurich University Hospital in Switzerland served as the stimulus for the incorporation of microvascular techniques in neurosurgery. In 1963, a 17-year-old girl awakened with hemiparesis after cardiac surgery. Left-sided carotid angiography revealed occlusion of the artery of the precentral gyrus. An emergency embolectomy was considered, but removal of the clot from such a small artery (0.8–1.1 mm) was technically impossible due to the lack of microsurgical skills and instruments. Fortunately, the patient improved over the course of several weeks, but the surgical staff's discussion about the need for microvascular techniques to approach lesions of the arteries of the cerebrum had a lasting impact.[8] Within 2 years, in 1965, a neurosurgeon from Zurich University Hospital who had been in practice for 11 years moved to Burlington to study microsurgical techniques under the supervision of Donaghy. The story of his training and his subsequent contributions to microsurgery are legendary. In 1999, this Turkish neurosurgeon, M. Gazi Yaşargil, was recognized as "Neurosurgery's Man of the Century 1950–1999" by the Congress of Neurological Surgeons.[9] Yaşargil developed his microsurgical skills by practicing on the peripheral arteries of dogs using 8–0 nylon sutures. After he completed 120 successful operations, he began practicing the same techniques on canine cerebral arteries, starting with the largest cerebral artery, the basilar artery.

Yaşargil soon found that the frontal and temporal cortical branches of the cerebral arteries were too small (0.4–0.6 mm) for the successful completion of anastomoses using 8–0 sutures. At first, only the basilar artery (1.0–1.2 mm) could be managed successfully with 8–0 sutures. However, in February 1966, bipolar coagulation (perfected by Leonard

Malis and introduced worldwide in 1955) became commercially available, which allowed Yaşargil to perform meticulous hemostasis. At the same time, new 9–0 sutures became available, which allowed Yaşargil to train on canine cerebral cortical vessels. Within a month, in March 1966, he completed the first successful extracranial-intracranial (EC-IC) anastomosis connecting the superficial temporal artery (STA) and the middle cerebral artery (MCA) in a dog.[10]

After his return to Zurich, Yaşargil performed the first STA-MCA bypass in an adult patient on October 30, 1967, only a day before Donaghy performed the same procedure in Vermont.[11] By 1968, a permanent laboratory for microsurgical training was established in Zurich. This commitment to extending and refining microsurgery techniques led to further advancements.

The decade of the 1970s saw similarly spectacular advancements in the field. In 1972, Yaşargil performed an EC-IC microanastomosis in a 4-year-old boy with moya-moya disease.[10] The positive outcome of that operation stimulated the further development of microsurgical methods for revascularization of the brain. Yaşargil is rightly considered to be the founder of what he eventually called "microneurosurgery," the specialty that applied microsurgery techniques to neurosurgery. His four-volume text, *Microneurosurgery*, remains a classic in the field.[12] About the same time, in 1971, William Lougheed and his team[13] published the results of the first high-flow bypass using a saphenous vein interpositional graft to connect the common carotid artery to the MCA.

During the early 1970s, the American neurosurgeon and neuroanatomist Albert L. Rhoton, Jr., established a microneurosurgical research center at the University of Florida.[14] His numerous publications on microneurosurgical anatomy have since become foundational classics throughout the world. Upon his death in 2016, an archive of his lifetime collection of neuroanatomy teaching materials (the Rhoton Collection) was made available free of charge worldwide.[15] Rhoton's legacy of clean, clear, illustrative, and educative neuroanatomical dissection techniques continues in the publications of many of Rhoton's fellows around the globe.

The following decades were characterized by the tempestuous and saltatory development of microsurgery across a range of surgical specialties. From an instrument of novelty in the 1960s and early 1970s, the microscope evolved into the most indispensable tool of the neurosurgeon. As microsurgery became an obligatory part of neurosurgery, clinical microsurgical training was integrated into educational programs in most United States, Japanese, and European neurosurgical centers. Today, it is difficult to imagine any neurosurgeon undertaking microsurgery on patients without first acquiring the basics of such training. This training can be optimized by the use of a specialized laboratory where most of the microsurgical operations can be practiced again and again. In the microsurgical laboratory, novice surgeons can familiarize themselves with the use of the microscope and the various microsurgical instruments. They can also study the principles and means of microsurgical interventions and continue to improve the skills they have obtained throughout their training. In many areas of neurosurgery, and also in other surgical specialties, microsurgical skills that have been developed and refined in the laboratory environment have a high degree of application to clinical practice.

Unfortunately, in many countries around the world, microsurgery is the only surgical specialty that makes microsurgical training obligatory for certification. Indeed, the existing number of specialized laboratories in universities and clinics would not be enough to support such a mandate. Thus, the individual surgeons who need such training—and the medical institutions that need such trained individuals—must tackle the crucial problem of developing the requisite microsurgical laboratories. To develop more qualified surgeons and to continue improving the quality of medical care for patients, each of us must tackle this problem by literally taking it into our own hands. We believe that surgeons can and will embrace this challenge and that neurosurgeons, in particular, are more than equal to the task. To that end, we have written this book to reflect the microsurgical training offered at our institutions in the hope that it will be a stepping stone for the development of similar programs elsewhere.

References

[1] Murphy JB. Resection of arteries and veins injured in continuity—end to end suture—experimental and clinical research. Med Rec (NY) 1897;51:73–88

[2] Carrel A. Landmark article, Nov 14, 1908: Results of the transplantation of blood vessels, organs and limbs. By Alexis Carrel. JAMA 1983;250(7):944–953

[3] Kurze T. Microtechniques in neurological surgery. Clin Neurosurg 1964;11:128–137

[4] Jacobson JH, Suarez EL. Microsurgery in anastomosis of small vessels. Surg Forum 1960;11:243

[5] Donalghy RMP, Yasargil MG. Micro-Vascular Surgery. Stuttgart: Georg Thieme Verlag; 1967

[6] Jacobson JH II, Wallman LJ, Schumacher GA, Flanagan M, Suarez EL, Donaghy RM. Microsurgery as an aid to middle cerebral artery endarterectomy. J Neurosurg 1962;19:108–115

[7] Fisher M. Occlusion of the internal carotid artery. AMA Arch Neurol Psychiatry 1951;65(3):346–377

[8] Yasargil MG. Remarks on the history or brain revascularization (foreword). In: Abdulrauf SI, ed. Remarks on the history or brain revascularization (foreword). Philadelphia: Saunders; 2011;XV–XXXVIII

[9] Yaşargil MG. A legacy of microneurosurgery: memoirs, lessons, and axioms. Neurosurgery 1999;45(5):1025–1092

[10] Yasargil MG. Microsurgery: Applied to Neurosurgery. New York, NY: Thieme; 2006

[11] Link TE, Bisson E, Horgan MA, Tranmer BI. Raymond M. P. Donaghy: a pioneer in microneurosurgery. J Neurosurg 2010;112(6):1176–1181

[12] Yasargil MG. Microneurosurgery. Stuttgart: Georg Thieme-Verlag; 1984

[13] Lougheed WM, Marshall BM, Hunter M, Michel ER, Sandwith-Smyth H. Common carotid to intracranial internal carotid bypass venous graft. Technical note. J Neurosurg 1971;34(1):114–118

[14] Friedman A. Albert L. Rhoton, Jr., M.D. World Neurosurg 2011;75(2):188–191, discussion 192–203

[15] Rutka JT. Editorial: The Rhoton Collection and the Journal of Neurosurgery: expanding the reach of neuroanatomy in the digital print world. J Neurosurg 2016;125(1):4–6

Acknowledgments

We are sincerely grateful to our teachers—including Robert F. Spetzler, Joseph M. Zabramski, and Mark C. Preul (Barrow Neurological Institute, Phoenix, Arizona); Ken-ichiro Kikuta (Fukui University, Fukui, Japan); Vadim A. Byvaltsev (Irkutsk State Medical University, Irkutsk, Russia); and Rosmarie Frick (University of Zurich, Zurich, Switzerland)—from whom we absorbed much knowledge and whose technical excellence in microsurgical techniques will remain an everlasting example for us to follow.

We thank the team of the Neuroscience Publications office of Barrow Neurological Institute, led by Mark Schornak. We are grateful to talented medical illustrators Peter M. Lawrence, Kristen Larson Keil, Jennifer Darcy, and Fiona Martin for transforming our ideas into beautiful and instructive illustrations. Many thanks to editorial assistants Samantha Soto and Rogena Lake for coordinating the preparation of this book and to production assistant Cindy Giljames for figure preparation. We are obliged to editors Dawn Mutchler and Joseph Mills and managing editors Mary Ann Clifft and Lynda Orescanin for thorough editing and numerous explanatory improvements. This book would have been incomplete without the support of Marie Clarkson, who edited the videos, and Gary Armstrong, who provided photographic and video equipment and helped to record the training.

We are also thankful to those companies and their representatives who provided instruments and equipment for the microsurgical training: Joshua Truitt (Mizuho America, Inc), Tony Bramblett (Kogent Surgical), Zach Edgmon (Aesculap, Inc), Brent Hartman (Medical Excellence Southwest), Jody Strauss (Medtronic, plc), Integra LifeSciences Corp, DePuy Synthes Companies, and Guido Hattendorf (Carl Zeiss Meditec AG).

Finally, and most importantly, we are deeply thankful to our families, whose loving support and patience allow us to devote our energy and time to our work.

Evgenii Belykh, MD
Nikolay L. Martirosyan, MD
M. Yashar S. Kalani, MD, PhD
Peter Nakaji, MD
Phoenix, Arizona

Contributors

Evgenii Belykh, MD, PhD
Neurosurgery Research Fellow
Department of Neurosurgery
Barrow Neurological Institute
Phoenix, Arizona
Assistant Professor
Department of Neurosurgery
Irkutsk State Medical University
Irkutsk, Russia

Vadim A. Byvaltsev, MD, PhD
Professor and Chairman
Department of Neurosurgery
Irkutsk State Medical University
Irkutsk, Russia

M. Yashar S. Kalani, MD, PhD
Vice Chair and Associate Professor
Director of Skull Base and Neurovascular Surgery
Departments of Neurosurgery and Neuroscience
University of Virginia School of Medicine
Charlottesville, Virginia

Ken-ichiro Kikuta, MD, PhD
Professor and Chairman
Department of Neurosurgery
Division of Medicine
Faculty of Medical Sciences
University of Fukui
Fukui, Japan

Nikolay L. Martirosyan, MD, PhD
Neurosurgery Fellow
Department of Neurosurgery
University of Arizona
Tucson, Arizona

Peter Nakaji, MD
Professor and Horace W. Steele Chair in Neurosurgical
   Innovation and Education
Program Director, Neurosurgery Residency Program
Barrow Neurological Institute
Phoenix, Arizona

Mark C. Preul, MD
Newsome Chair and Director of Neurosurgery Research
Director, The Loyal and Edith Davis Neurosurgical Research
   Laboratory
Professor of Neurosurgery and Neuroscience
Department of Neurosurgery
Barrow Neurological Institute
Phoenix, Arizona

Robert F. Spetzler, MD
Emeritus President and CEO of Barrow Neurological
   Institute
Emeritus Chair
Department of Neurosurgery
Barrow Neurological Institute
Phoenix, Arizona

1 The Philosophy of Microsurgical Practice: Four Founding Principles Inherited from the Great Thinkers

Evgenii Belykh and Peter Nakaji

Abstract

The philosophy of microsurgical training is underpinned by four essential principles: (1) close replication of the microsurgery environment results in familiarity and ease with actual procedures; (2) repeated practice of the same techniques builds muscle memory and enhances mindfulness; (3) thoughtful preparation and rehearsal; and (4) training on increasingly more complex microsurgical tasks builds higher level skill and aids progress through the stages of competence. These principles encompass the essence of how well-planned, deliberate, thorough, and repeated microneurosurgical practice within a laboratory setting can improve the operative skill set of the neurosurgeon. Such training facilitates the refinement of the manual skills needed by neurosurgeons not only to enhance their professional ability but also to treat their future patients, whose welfare rests in their hands.

Keywords: anastomosis, bypass, competence, deliberate practice, mindfulness, movements, philosophy, practice, training

1.1 Introduction

Cerebrovascular surgeries are challenging and may be viewed as battles of a neurosurgeon against the pathology, with the battlefield being the most complex and precious area of the body—the human brain. Our way of thinking about and preparing for complex cerebrovascular surgeries and bypass procedures in particular, interestingly, is in line with classical philosophical teachings. At its finest, the art of microsurgery is an endeavor illustrating the pinnacle of human skill. Guiding principles borrowed from the military strategist and philosopher Sun Tzu, Taoism philosopher and moralist Chuang Tzŭ, and innovator and pioneer in industrialization Henry Ford underpin our view on the philosophy of microsurgical training. The following four principles will help to navigate the trainee through microsurgical training and form a framework that can aid in the production of better trained, more confident, and more competent neurosurgeons.

1.2 Principle One: The Terrain

"The natural formation of the country is the soldier's best ally."

—Sun Tzu

The trainee should always seek to expand his or her understanding of the landscape of microsurgical approaches. Our mind is limited by conceptions of what is possible and what is not possible in a particular clinical situation, what is acceptable and what is unacceptable, and what is reversible and what is irreversible. Most of the limits in our mind are psychological, practical, economic, or aesthetic in nature and are flexible, while others, like physiological and anatomical boundaries, are more rigid. However, even technical and physiological boundaries that are perceived as absolute are mostly due to the gaps in our knowledge of surgical anatomy or lack of awareness of new techniques or technologies. There are many neurosurgical centers that have various visions relating to the uses and utility of cerebrovascular bypasses. Still, the first principle, the knowledge of neuroanatomy, remains perpetual and foundational. Understanding of natural "narrow passes," "accessible grounds," safe zones, and the normal and pathological locations of the vasculature grants the surgeon confidence and creates comfortable terrain for work with cerebral arteries and for performing bypasses in the service of the treatment of cerebrovascular diseases.

The environment and models for microsurgical training ideally should be as close to real conditions as possible, especially during the final stages of training. This facility with simulated surgery allows the trainee to face challenges and take advantage of the terrain presented by patients' anatomy in performing microsurgical approaches.

1.3 Principle Two: The Movement

"A deal of poverty grows out of the carriage of excess weight."

—Henry Ford

Dynamic stereotypes developed in our unconscious minds are potentially more powerful than those in our conscious minds. Complex, rapid, and accurate instrument manipulation in the hand of an expert neurosurgeon constitutes a dynamic stereotype that can be divided into several simpler acts or moves. Many movements, especially for the early trainee, are inefficient; they have "excess weight" that makes the performance "poor." Creating a new dynamic stereotype for microsurgery is difficult, but unlearning old, inefficient stereotypes is sometimes even more difficult. Learning a new, efficient, dynamic stereotype requires disassembly of the old stereotype and stepwise assembly of a new one.

For neurosurgeons who will specialize in microsurgery, frequent and repeated practice in the laboratory will ingrain the specialized habits required for microanastomosis so that the individual steps of an operation can be done by rote, without hesitation. With repeated practice of separate steps, the subconscious soon realizes what must be delivered to meet the desired goals. As these steps blend together, the process becomes increasingly fluid, which allows the surgeon to concentrate on higher level functions: the conscious mind of the surgeon is free to focus on decision-making and adapting the procedure to the particular needs of the individual patient, as dictated by anatomy and the clinical situation.

Having done the necessary work to make the basic processes of microsurgery comfortable and automatic allows the surgeon

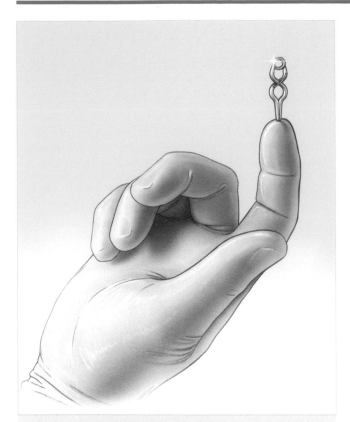

Fig. 1.1 Balancing an aneurysm clip on the tip of the finger. An artistic metaphor for the complete concentration and accuracy required for mastering microneurosurgery.

overall surgical skill set. Few if any would question this assertion, which is supported by ample evidence.[3,4]

Accurately and rapidly anastomosing the thinnest and smallest of blood vessels in the human brain is a daunting endeavor and should be regarded with appropriate gravity. Dissecting the perforators off the dome of a ruptured aneurysm is an act of fortitude and precision conducted a fraction of a millimeter away from human tragedy. Yet these and other microsurgical techniques are much more than mere physical acts. Just as peak athletic performance is as much mental as it is physical, microsurgery also requires a mindset that is developed by years of rigorous discipline and preparation, calm equanimity, and mindfulness. The microsurgery operating suite has no room for anxiety, distraction, or agitation. The surgeon must be completely present and fully aware.

Extensive practice leads to a high level of reproducibility, which yields superior results that, in turn, build confidence and create an upward spiral of success.

1.5 Principle Four: Complete the "Four Stages of the Fighting Rooster"

"Chi Hsing Tzǔ was training fighting cocks for the prince.
At the end of ten days the latter asked if they were ready. 'Not yet', replied Chi; 'they are in the stage of seeking fiercely for a foe'.
Again ten days elapsed, and the prince made a further enquiry. 'Not yet', replied Chi; 'they are still excited by the sounds and shadows of other cocks'.
Ten days more, and the prince asked again. 'Not yet', answered Chi; 'the sight of an enemy is still enough to excite them to rage'.
But after another ten days, when the prince again enquired, Chi said, 'They will do. Other cocks may crow, but they will take no notice. To look at them one might say they were of wood. Their virtue is complete. Strange cocks will not dare meet them, but will run'."

—Chuang Tzǔ

Any new skill develops through four main stages: unconscious incompetence, conscious incompetence, conscious competence, and finally unconscious competence (▶ Fig. 1.2).[6] Awareness of these stages helps individuals to understand their personal position on the learning curve and to visualize the skills that they will need to acquire in their career several years ahead. They can thereby anticipate possible mistakes and be prepared mentally for the arduous process of complex microsurgical skill acquisition. Concordant with the views of contemporary psychology, these four stages of skill acquisition are nicely illustrated by the ancient Chinese parable about the training of the fighting rooster.[5,7]

In the first stage, the trainee knows the strokes and techniques of a microanastomosis and even performs it decently on the mannequin. The trainee often thinks that he/she is ready to perform the procedure on patients in every situation. However, the trainee has not experienced the real conditions of surgery. In imaginary battles, the trainee wins imaginary victories. The trainee may not care who or what the patient is, as all cases look similar.

to relax mentally and physically and thereby to experience less personal stress, which by extension will ease the inherent stress of the operation for the support staff (▶ Fig. 1.1). A more relaxed operating team works together more smoothly and dispatches minor irregularities in the procedure with ease.

1.4 Principle Three: The Preparation

"The general who wins the battle makes many calculations in his temple before the battle is fought. The general who loses makes but few calculations beforehand."

—Sun Tzu

Achieving a heightened state of mindfulness does not come simply from believing in it or willing it. It is a state gained through disciplined practice. Yet the fundamental skills of microsurgery should not be developed and acquired while working on patients. The neurosurgeon should emulate the musical performer, who does not make an audience endure endless rehearsals, or the bomb squad that defuses live bombs only after practicing endlessly on fake ones. The neurosurgeon should refine and maintain these skills through practice in preparation for surgery on patients. As Anders Ericsson and colleagues[1,2] have noted, deliberate practice improves performance in the individual operation being practiced and strengthens one's

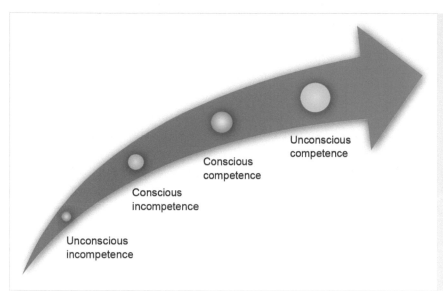

Fig. 1.2 Diagram of skill development stages.

In the second stage, the trainee may grow concerned due to the experience of suffering defeats in real surgeries. The trainee understands that the consequences of surgical actions are meaningful and that many complications are hard to foresee.

In the third stage, the trainee has real victories and procedural successes. However, the trainee is still subject to conflicting emotions of disappointment and a desire for courage, which has a noticeable effect on performance. When the "fight" takes all the surgeon's concentration, other factors can intrude that go unnoticed and may still ruin the battle.

In the fourth stage, the surgeon is calm and unemotional. His or her image speaks for him or her. The skills and instrument movements look effortlessly natural and intuitive. The trainee, now a master, has already beaten the opponent with his or her calm mind. However, it should be noted that, behind the intuitive and adroit surgical moves, there are many small but critical factors that are responding to details of the surgical field, which we begin to appreciate only with experience.

To earn the trust of patients enough to be allowed to perform microsurgical work on their brains—arguably the very seat of the soul—the surgeon must complete whatever preparation is necessary to be worthy of the honor. This means completing long hours of dedicated study, intellectually mastering indications and techniques, and spending as much time as needed to achieve technical familiarity, facility, refinement, and, finally, mastery of the techniques. This process is never ending, and mastering the four stages may reflect a lifetime of career experience. We have a moral and ethical obligation not just to learn but also to keep learning and to drive the field forward, until that day in the distant future when advances in medicine may make such skills obsolete.

References

[1] Ericsson KA. Acquisition and maintenance of medical expertise: a perspective from the expert-performance approach with deliberate practice. Acad Med; 90(11):1471–1486

[2] Crochet P, Aggarwal R, Dubb SS, et al. Deliberate practice on a virtual reality laparoscopic simulator enhances the quality of surgical technical skills. Ann Surg; 253(6):1216–1222

[3] Gélinas-Phaneuf N, Del Maestro RF. Surgical expertise in neurosurgery: integrating theory into practice. Neurosurgery; 73 Suppl 1:30–38

[4] van de Wiel MW, Van den Bossche P, Janssen S, Jossberger H. Exploring deliberate practice in medicine: how do physicians learn in the workplace? Adv Health Sci Educ Theory Pract; 16(1):81–95

[5] Tzŭ C. Chuang Tzŭ. Giles HA, transl. London: Bernard Quaritch; 1889

[6] Kavis M. The Four Stages of Cloud Competence. 2015. Available at: https://www.forbes.com/sites/mikekavis/2015/10/21/the-four-stages-of-cloud-competence/#3382fb1c183a. Accessed September 2010 and 2017

[7] Tarasov V. Art of Management Fighting. Tallinn: Kvibek Trade; 2002

2 Day 1: The Organization of the Microsurgical Laboratory: Necessary Tools and Equipment

Evgenii Belykh, Nikolay L. Martirosyan, and Mark C. Preul

Abstract

The organization of the microneurosurgical training laboratory is essential to an effective neurosurgical training program. In this chapter, we review key organizational aspects, list the necessary equipment, and discuss principal microneurosurgical instruments.

Keywords: exoscope, forceps, microsurgical laboratory setup, microscissors, microsurgical instruments, operative microscope

2.1 Organization of the Microsurgical Training Laboratory

The microsurgical laboratory should be headed by a qualified neurosurgeon who has microsurgical experience, who can provide oversight and guidance for such work, and who has an established record of service and rapport with trainees. Work in the modern microsurgical laboratory can range from training only with artificial materials to working with biological materials (e.g., animal and human placentas), cadaveric tissues, and animals. Training exercises that involve more than artificial materials will require appropriate facilities, staff, and institutional approvals and inspections, especially for the use of live animals or cadaveric tissues as a part of the training.

Because the activities of the laboratory center on learning specific neurosurgical techniques or maneuvers, these are best coordinated by the neurosurgical department of the sponsoring hospital or university. Most laboratories allow shared access to the facilities by various clinical and educational departments in different specialties. Allowing 24-hour access (including on weekends) helps to make the microsurgical practice opportunities available to as many busy specialists as possible, which maximizes the use of expensive microscope and laboratory resources. Ideally, a coordinating administrator will design a well-defined program and training schedule for the trainees. As interns or junior residents master their basic microsurgical skills, they are not yet performing the corresponding operations in patients, and they may continue their education and practice their skills during more flexible hours.[1,2,3,4] Even experienced neurosurgeons will benefit from performing "off-the-job training" to maintain their microsurgical skills.[5] Such ongoing practice increases efficiency in an operating room and raises the incidence of technical success.[6] It has been suggested that a neurosurgeon needs at least 10,000 hours of training, including on decision-making, to become competent, confident, and technically skilled.[7]

2.2 Laboratory Setup

Ideally, the laboratory should be set up away from the clinical departments in its own space near the vivarium. Because of regulations and the obvious potential for contamination from animal, cadaveric, and other biological tissues, training activities using these materials must be isolated from patient care areas. A well-outfitted bioskills laboratory also has operating rooms and conference rooms within the same facility. The conference room should include a library (with microsurgical videos, books, and articles) equipped with computer workstations that provide access to the medical literature and have servers for data storage. Such a facility may be difficult to establish, given the already high demand for research space in many medical institutions. At a minimum, the goal should be to designate an area where the trainee will be undisturbed and will have access to the appropriate instruments and visualization, including an operative microscope, to perform the required procedures.

The ideal operating room in a practice laboratory is a space with an area of more than 20 square meters (just over 215 square feet), in an illuminated, well-ventilated room equipped with a microscope with excellent optical performance and an operative table. Surgical chairs should be placed in such a way that two people (trainer and trainee) can perform each exercise together opposite to each other. Optimally, the surgical chairs should be the same type used in the operating room. The chairs should be comfortable, should have armrests, and should be able to have the height adjusted. A sink with a water supply system and a basin for washing and cleaning (i.e., sanitizing) instruments is essential. The special sterilization equipment and sterile space necessary for research projects involving survival experiments are not routinely needed for training purposes involving animal sacrifice (▶ Fig. 2.1). Ideally, the laboratory should have storage for biological tissues used for training, such as a dedicated refrigerator and freezer, and cabinets for formaldehyde-preserved specimens.

The ethical and responsible conduct of research and training in the laboratory should be followed by all trainees who work and train in the laboratory. The laboratory staff and trainees should complete regular certification courses (online Collaborative Institutional Training Initiative [CITI] training or equivalent) on biosafety and biosecurity, on responsible conduct of research, and on animal care and use. In most instances, the trainee should also be briefly instructed by a local veterinarian before working with animals.

Because it contains expensive equipment and instruments, the laboratory should support an appropriate level of electronic security and should be kept locked when not in use. Only approved personnel should have access to the laboratory. Residents and other trainees should be in constant contact with the staff and manager of the laboratory to make sure that lost and damaged instruments are replaced.

2.3 Materials and Equipment

To effectively perform microsurgical operations, even in practice sessions, neurosurgeons must have at least a minimal set of essential equipment. The essentials include an operative microscope, microsurgical instruments, and suture material. Any instrument used in microsurgery training should meet the technical conditions required for those used in clinical surgery. When the quality of the microsurgical instruments used in training is as high as that of those used in clinical surgery, the training will prepare the neurosurgeon better for actual surgery. The main types of equipment used in the training laboratory are the operative microscope, surgical loupes, exoscope, microsurgical instruments (needle holder, forceps, scissors, vascular clips, clip applier, scalpel), bipolar coagulation, retractors, irrigator and solutions for irrigation, suction devices and suction cannulas, sponges and gauze, sutures and needles, dyes,

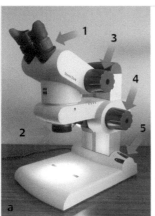

Fig. 2.1 Microsurgical bypass workstation in the Neurosurgery Research Laboratory, Department of Neurosurgery, Barrow Neurological Institute, Phoenix, Arizona.

background material, high-speed drill, and various stimulation devices.

2.3.1 Operative Microscopes

Optimally, the training operative microscope should be the same as or similar to the type of microscope used in surgery. Efficient manipulation of the modern operative microscope requires some training, so similarity allows the trainee to build skills that will translate more smoothly to the operating suite. The principal structure of the microscope resembles that of the microscopes that many students use in high school or college biology classes, with some important differences. The main parts of the microscope are shown in ▶ Fig. 2.2.

The trainee must be able to adjust and confidently operate the microscope. Most neurosurgery is performed under substantial magnification (within the range of 4x to 40x). Thus, a byproduct of practicing surgical hand skills in the neurosurgical training laboratory should be the attainment of familiarity and expertise with working in a magnified anatomical environment.

The operative microscope should be firmly affixed to the table or it should have a heavy base with a hard platform to hold it steady and minimize oscillations. Modern microscopes have a built-in computer with dedicated software that controls the positioning of the microscope head and the camera that records video. The working head of the microscope includes a main objective lens and a magnification changer directed at the operative field, two sets of binocular eyepieces for the surgeon and the surgical assistant with switchable positions, and handgrips with multiple programmable buttons to release and reposition the microscope, change focus and magnification, start and stop video recording, and activate fluorescence (▶ Fig. 2.3). Operative microscopes are also equipped with a portable foot control panel (also called foot pedal or foot switch) with programmable buttons and functions similar to the handgrips.

Modern operative microscopes have an electric motor that affords smooth movements for repositioning the microscope. A well-balanced microscope head can be moved in multiple directions with handgrips, a foot control panel, or a mouth

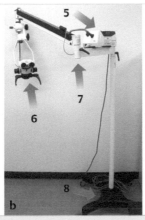
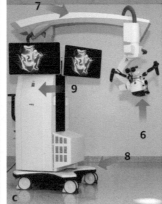
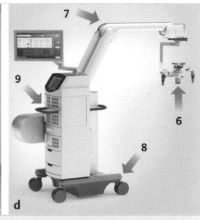

Fig. 2.2 Modern microscopes: **(a)** the STEMI DV4 laboratory-grade benchtop stereomicroscope (Carl Zeiss, Inc.), **(b)** a Leica operative microscope (Leica Microsystems, GmbH), **(c)** a Zeiss operative microscope (Kinevo 900, Carl Zeiss Meditec AG, Inc.), and **(d)** the HS 5–1000 operative microscope system (Haag-Streit Surgical). 1, eyepieces; 2, objective lens; 3, zoom adjustment knob; 4, focal distance adjustment knob; 5, light controller; 6, working head; 7, movable arm; 8, base; and 9, built-in computer. (Figs. 2.2a, b are provided courtesy of Evgenii Belykh, MD. Fig. 2.2d is used with permission from Haag-Streit, USA.)

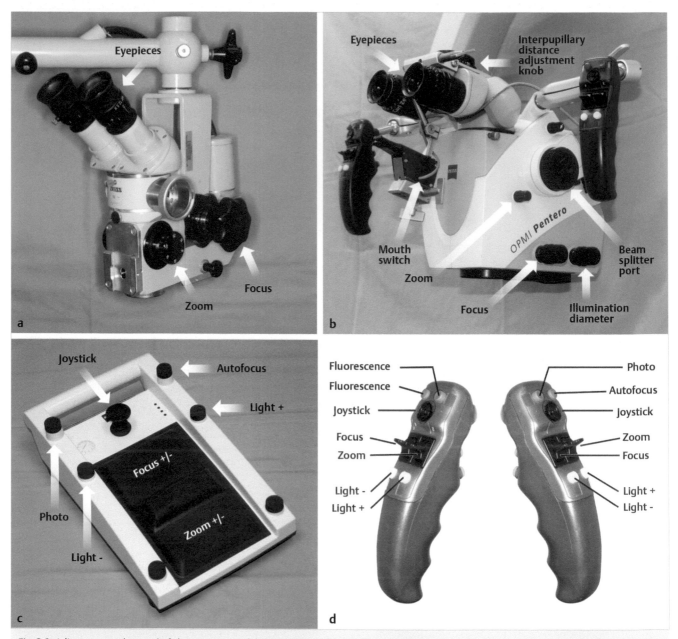

Fig. 2.3 Adjustment and control of the microscope. (a) Zeiss OPMI 1, (b) Zeiss Pentero, (c) foot control panel, and (d) handgrip with the buttons programmed as preferred by Dr. Robert F. Spetzler. Note that eyepieces have diopter adjustment rings and soft eyecups, with adjustable length.

switch (▶ Fig. 2.4). Although not included with the standard microscope configuration, a headpiece device for the surgeon has been developed that allows hands-free positioning of the microscope.[8] The surgeon's and face-to-face observer's microscopic views are three-dimensional because of the two space-separated beams of light projecting in two eyepieces separately (▶ Fig. 2.5). However, the side observer's view is not three-dimensional because both observers eyepieces receive the same one beam of light from a side beam splitter (▶ Fig. 2.5). The operative field is illuminated coaxially through the objective lens from a built-in light source. Coaxial lighting is absolutely essential for reaching deep lesions; thus, it is also needed in training exercises involving a deep operative field.

Despite the complex structure of the various types of modern microscopes, the principles of working with them remain the same. The basic adjustments of the microscope for obtaining an optimal view include adjustment of (1) the interpupillary distance of the eyepieces; (2) the individual eyepiece magnification with the diopter setting ring for sight correction; (3) the zoom (magnification); and (4) the focal distance, either manually (basic models) or automatically (advanced models).

The surgeon sets the appropriate *interpupillary distance* by positioning his or her eyes about 1 inch from the eyepiece. The small round optical fields should be visible separately. The adjusting knob is then turned until the two circles overlap completely. Most microscopes have an interpupillary distance scale near the knob for fast settings. With repeated practice, trainees

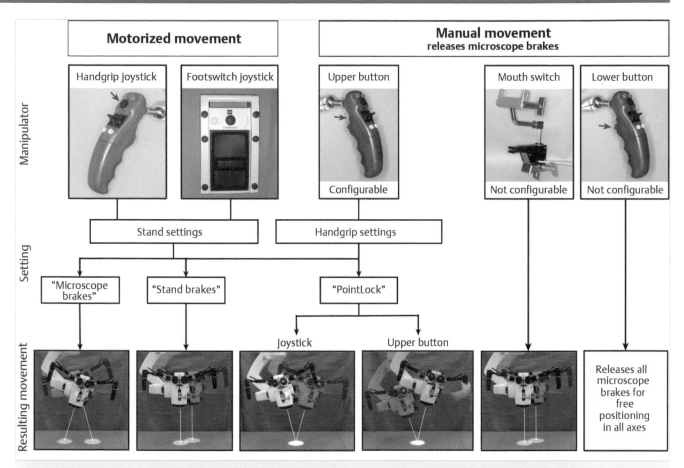

Fig. 2.4 Schematic of possible ways to control movement of the robotic operative microscope (Kinevo 900, Carl Zeiss Meditec AG). Movement can be either motorized or manual. The control for the various settings can be assigned to buttons and joysticks on the handgrips and footswitch; the mouth switch and the lower button on the handgrip are not configurable.

will begin to remember the exact value of their own interpupillary distance.

The *eyepiece diopter correction* is essential for maintaining the focus of the microscope whenever the magnification is changed. If the operator needs no correction for his or her vision, the eyepiece should be set at zero. Nearsighted or farsighted operators who wish to operate without glasses should adjust the diopter setting of the eyepiece according to their individual eyeglasses prescription. Alternatively, the microscope can be used while wearing eyeglasses, especially if the correction is more than 3 diopters. When using eyeglasses, the eyecaps on the eyepieces should be adjusted to a minimum to ensure the full field of view is visible. On some microscopes, the rubber eyecup should be removed from the eyepieces in order to see the full field of view when wearing eyeglasses.

The *focal distance* of the microscope lens is one of its most important features. In older models of the operative microscope and in the most current laboratory-grade stereomicroscopes, the total focal distance is significantly affected by the focal distance of the objective lens. In such microscopes, the focal distance is indicated on the frame of the lens, and it must correspond to the distance between the lens and the planned surgical target. Objective lenses are available with various focal distances (e.g., 200 mm, 250 mm, 300 mm, 400 mm, etc.) and can be interchanged before surgery to accommodate longer

(~40–50 cm in spine surgery) and shorter (~20–40 cm in cranial surgery) working distances. Most modern operative microscopes incorporate a variable focusing system (varioscope) that allows for continuous adjustment of the working distance and magnification for near distance positioning and for far distance positioning, without the need to change the objective lens.

The total *magnification* of the microscope depends on the focal distance of the objective lens and on the magnification factor of the three key optical components: the eyepieces, the magnification changer, and the objective lens (▶ Fig. 2.6). Eyepieces usually have a magnification of 10x or 12.5x for operative microscopes, although higher magnifications (20x) may be chosen for custom-built training stereomicroscopes.

The magnification changer assemblies of operative microscopes differ significantly from those of laboratory stereomicroscopes. Depending on the configuration of the operative microscope, the magnification changer assembly may include up to three components for magnification adjustment: a foldable binocular tube with an integrated two-step manual magnification changer (Promag [Carl Zeiss Meditec, Inc.], 1.0x or 1.5x magnification); an additional three-step manual magnification changer (1x, 0.6x, and 1.6x); and a motorized zoom lens mechanism. The zoom lens mechanism provides a stepless change of magnification from 0.4x to 2.4x. The field of view diameter depends on the magnification and is between 1 and 10 cm.

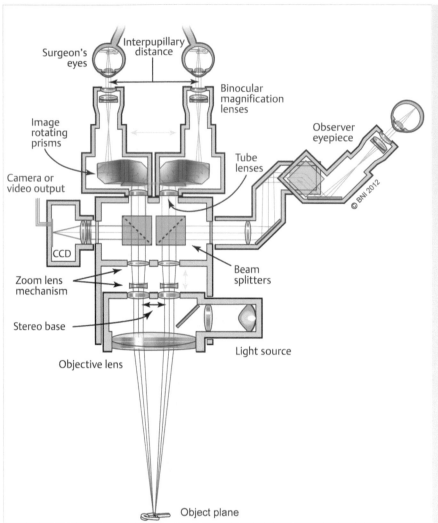

Fig. 2.5 Artist's illustration demonstrating the lighting pathway and optics of the operative microscope.

The *field of clear view* (i.e., the *focal depth*) is the range of depth of the operative wound that is clearly visible at a given distance through the microscope. This depth depends on the focal distance of the lens, the degree of magnification, and the optical system of the microscope. In modern microscopes, the field of clear view is deep enough to provide a clear and in-focus view of both deep and shallow structures in the surgical landscape. The focal distance must be adjusted such that most of the field of clear view is slightly higher than the object, which allows the surgeon to clearly see the tips of the instruments and the operative field. The surgeon should first adjust the focus to the highest magnification and then return the setting to the lower magnification. Doing so allows the object to remain in focus when the magnification is subsequently changed. This algorithm for adjusting the microscope is essential knowledge for any trainee (▶ Table 2.1).

Control of light intensity and magnification are essential for microscopes used in training. The most suitable microscopes for laboratory use have a built-in white light source (typically halogen), a magnification of 2x to 40x, and a focal distance of 200 to 400 mm. The training microscope should also have a double optical system or a built-in video camera connected to a monitor to enable the instructor and the trainee to observe each other's technique. This system enables the instructor to coach the trainee and to evaluate the trainee's skills.

The use of video recording can facilitate the post-training assessment of the technique. It allows trainees to film their microsurgical practice sessions for self-analysis and for later discussion with the instructor. Videos from practice sessions can be used to capture photographs, which can be used for publications. In addition, intraoperative images can form the basis for artist's illustrations.

A portable benchtop stereomicroscope is suitable for initial and continuing dry microsurgical training (▶ Fig. 2.2a). However, unless they are customized, benchtop stereomicroscopes usually have a short focal distance that does not allow training with long instruments in a deep operative field. In contrast, simple operative microscopes, such as OPMI 1 (Carl Zeiss Meditec, Inc.) and higher-grade microscopes, have a longer focal length and a flexible suspension system and are considered optimal for a training laboratory (▶ Fig. 2.2b–d).

In some ways, the surgeon can be compared to a fighter pilot, who must study the operation of the aircraft engine in order to become intimately familiar with it, even if someone else performs the actual engine maintenance. Learning the proper operation, care, and maintenance of the microscope is part of the

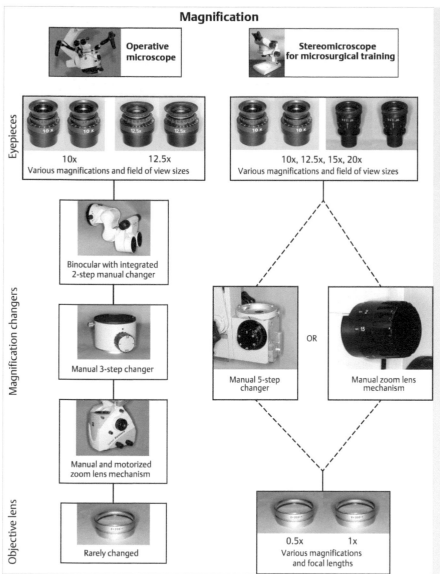

Fig. 2.6 Schematic of the optical parts of an operative microscope used for magnification adjustment. Left column: parts of the operative microscope that must be adjusted appropriately during surgery; right column: optical parts of a custom stereomicroscope used for microsurgical training. A combination of a long-focal-distance, low-magnification objective lens (0.5x) with high-magnification eyepieces (20x) can increase the working distance and make the laboratory stereomicroscope suitable for microsurgical training with long shaft instruments, while continuing to have high magnification. (ZEISS Stemi 305 photograph is licensed under the Creative Commons Attribution-Share Alike 2.0 Generic license.)

Table 2.1 Method for adjusting the microscope to achieve a constant sharp image throughout the entire magnification

Start this procedure for adjustment of one eyepiece	
1	Position the microscope above a flat object at a working distance of 20–25 cm
2	Set the microscope to the lowest magnification
3	Adjust diopter setting ring on eyepiece to 0 diopters
4	Look through the eyepiece and focus image sharply
5	Set the microscope to the highest magnification and correct the fine focusing until the image is sharp
6	Set the microscope back to the lowest magnification without changing the working distance
7	Adjust the diopter setting ring on the eyepiece to the maximum positive value (+ 5 diopters)
8	Look through the eyepiece and slowly turn the diopter setting ring in the minus diopter direction until the image is once again defined sharply
Repeat the entire procedure for the second eyepiece	
Source: Adapted from Kinevo manual, Carl Zeiss Meditec AG.	

surgeon's job, simply because the microscope is such an essential part of the operating room armamentarium. Preoperatively, the surgeon should check three important systems of the microscope: the electrical, mechanical, and optical systems. The electrical components include the manipulators, the foot control panel, and the light source. The handgrips and the foot control panel should be tested to ensure that the microscope will respond to their commands. Buttons and switches on the handgrips and foot control panel should be programmed beforehand in the way that is most comfortable for the neurosurgeon (▶ Fig. 2.3c,d, ▶ Fig. 2.4). If the microscope light is not bright enough or if the remaining lamp life is short (based on the total hours used, usually 500 h maximum), it should be replaced beforehand to prevent the loss of illumination during a critical step of the operation. Other checks include the proper positioning of the microscope in the operating room, the proper placement of the eyepieces for the surgical assistant, and the balancing of the microscope head to ensure its smooth and easy movement. Finally, all the lenses should be cleaned, especially the objective lens, which often becomes soiled by droplets of blood and solutions. Any necessary optical adjustments can be made to the lenses after they are cleaned.

Setting Up the Operative Microscope

When preparing the operative microscope for use, the following sequence should be observed:

1. Change the objective lens to one with a focal distance (f) that corresponds to the distance from the microscope to the operative field. Typically, a lens with $f = 20$ cm is used for surface operations, one with $f = 40$ cm is used for spinal surgery, and one with $f = 30$ cm is used for cranial operations.
2. Position the co-observation tube for the surgical assistant in accordance with the operation: face to face (for spine and microsurgery training) or to the side beam splitter port (for cranial and microsurgery training). The side is usually opposite to the hemisphere being operated, that is, the co-observation tube will be on the left for a right-sided approach.
3. Check the functionality of all the electrical, mechanical, and optical parts of the microscope, including the knobs and electronic switches that control the light, magnification, focus, and release of the magnetic brakes.
4. Balance the microscope.
5. Adjust the interpupillary distance of the eyepieces.
6. Adjust the eyecup so the entire field of view is visible.
7. Adjust the diopter setting on the eyepieces separately for each eye.
8. Set the microscope to the lowest magnification.
9. Cover the microscope with a sterile drape.

2.3.2 Surgical Loupes

Unlike high-cost microscopes (that may cost anywhere from US $10,000–$500,000), surgical loupes (that usually cost from US $20$1,000) are a cheaper and more mobile instrument. However, surgical loupes are not adjustable and they lack the necessary magnification to support many microsurgical manipulations. They provide only low-resolution views (the usual magnification is 2x to 8x), which make it difficult to maintain a

clear view during some manipulations. Loupes can have either a fixed working distance or an adjustable working distance (the distance between the eyes and the operational field). Before purchasing personal loupes, surgeons should determine their individual optimal working distance. Although loupes are considered a personal item, those with adjustable intrapupillary distance can be shared by several users, which can be economically advantageous.

2.3.3 Exoscopes

The exoscope is another technologically advanced tool in the surgeon's armamentarium that is used to provide a magnified view of the operative field. The exoscope combines the features of an endoscope and a microscope. The optics of the exoscope are positioned outside of the wound, like a microscope, but the image is displayed on a monitor similar to the way an endoscope functions. Exoscopes display high-quality two-dimensional or three-dimensional video with acceptable visualization of the surgical field and a wide range of magnification from 2x to 40x. (▶ Fig. 2.7). Exoscopic technologies are only now being integrated into operating room equipment used by neurosurgeons but will likely be routinely used alongside the operative microscope in the near future.[9,10] Some exoscopes have a robotic positioning arm that automatically aligns the exoscope with the desired trajectory by using neuronavigation input or by using controls on the foot pedal. This hands-free positioning function presents a completely new way of providing visualization in the operating room, which increases the surgeon's

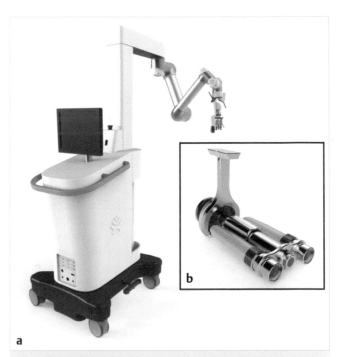

Fig. 2.7 Exoscope technology combines the visualization power of an operative microscope with the flexibility and ergonomics of a small video camera. The operator sees an image of the operative field on the monitor that is the same as the one seen through the endoscope. **(a)** Unit, monitor, and robotic arm; and **(b)** exoscope optical lens and illumination lights. (Used with permission from Synaptive Medical, Inc.)

comfort when working on deep structures within narrow and complex anatomical corridors. Our laboratory experience with the exoscope indicates that its combination of high magnification with a high-resolution stereoscopic view facilitates the performance of microsurgical steps, with technical results comparable to those with the use of a standard operative microscope.

2.3.4 Microsurgical Instruments

The ability to properly perform microsurgical techniques depends not only on the extent of the surgeon's training, but also on the quality of the instruments the surgeon uses. The actual effects of surgery are actuated by the use of the microsurgical instruments, so the better the instruments, the better the microsurgical results. The extremely thin tips of the instruments can be easily bent, making it impossible for them to properly hold suture materials and tissues. Having to work with damaged instruments—even during microsurgical practice—can create unnecessary difficulties, frustration, and anxiety. The end result is often a lesson on how not to perform better; instead, the surgeon or trainee must focus only on how to overcome the obstacles that might otherwise have been easily prevented. Thus, trying to practice with less than perfect microinstruments is simply a waste of precious time. There is no nobility in working with bad instruments, even in the laboratory.

Ideally, each trainee should have a personal set of microsurgical instruments, with a customized case and rack for them. Each trainee should also have an individual microscope, or an assigned and protected time to work with the laboratory microscope during training. In some neurosurgical centers in Japan, the United States, and China, trainees are provided with personal microsurgical instruments that are paid for by the clinic or university. However, the high cost of microsurgical instruments precludes such largesse in every case. Thus, the training laboratory should always have on hand several sets of the basic microinstruments for common use. Microsurgical instruments produced by different companies differ greatly in quality and price. We recommend nonmagnetic titanium or high-grade stainless steel corrosion-proof microsurgical instruments.[11]

In choosing the microsurgical instruments they will use, surgeons should pay attention to the shape of the handle, because the shape influences the surgeon's ability to manipulate the instrument as needed without losing control of it. Most handle shapes are either flat or round. Instruments with a bayonet-like shape are used for microsurgery in a deep and narrow operative wound. Bayoneted instruments prevent the hand and the handle from overlapping with the microscopic field of view during surgical maneuvers. Most instruments have fluted or corrugated surfaces on the handles to increase friction and resistance to slipping. With increasing experience, each neurosurgeon develops his or her own preferences regarding the types of instruments and the methods for holding them.

One of the most important characteristics of microsurgical instruments is their fragility. The tip of an instrument can be measured in thousandths of an inch, which corresponds to the thickness of the 10–0 suture. Following several simple rules will keep instruments in perfect condition for a long time:

1. Do not transport an instrument outside the case, which makes it more vulnerable to being bent if it is accidentally dropped. Always transport the instruments in the carrying case, whether they are dirty or clean.
2. Do not hold more than one instrument in one hand.
3. Always clean the instruments one by one.
4. Do not mix microsurgical instruments with other surgical instruments.
5. Do not touch the tips of the microsurgical instruments to other hard metal objects.
6. To avoid rust, do not keep the instruments moist for a long time or autoclave the instruments far in advance of use.
7. Do not use the instruments for work on cadavers or other non-living biological tissues, because by regulation they must be cleaned and stored separately from instruments used in survival animal surgery. All instruments used in survival animal surgery must be sterile.

Following these simple rules will help to maintain the microsurgical instruments in perfect condition over a longer period of time. Doing so will also lead to a better training experience and will facilitate many surgeries.

Needle Holders

The needle holder is optional for microneurosurgical training, because in most cases a needle can be handled with forceps. Many neurosurgeons use microforceps as needle holders, partly because it rules out the necessity of choosing the proper instrument to perform surgical manipulations between suturing. Needle holders come with and without a locking mechanism. Locking needle holders are not used for microsurgery, because their tips shift when the locking mechanism is opened or closed. Standard small stainless steel microsurgical needle holders with curved tips are good enough for initial microsurgical training (▶ Fig. 2.8). The sole advantage of needle holders over microforceps is the solid fixation of the needle. However, in some cases, the use of a needle holder can be advantageous. For example, a needle holder with long rounded handles and curved tips (▶ Fig. 2.8e) might be particularly useful for performing anastomosis in a deep and narrow operative corridor.

Forceps

Microforceps are mandatory for training and clinical practice. They can be purchased in different sizes, with different tip shapes and handle styles, and made of different materials (▶ Fig. 2.9, ▶ Fig. 2.10). Microforceps are used to hold sutures, needles, and tissues. They are also used to tie knots. These thin-tip forceps (tips of 0.1 to 0.2 mm diameter) are essential for working with vessels whose diameter is 1 mm or less. Microforceps should be reserved for the handling of the most delicate tissues. They should not be used during the gross stages of an operation, even on experimental animals, because the tips may bend or become deformed in other ways.

Knot-Tying Forceps

Knot-tying forceps have a flat platform (▶ Fig. 2.10c) and slightly raised tips to facilitate the grasping and holding of sutures. This platform allows the tips to close evenly over several tenths of a millimeter without excessive pressure, which enables smooth and easy knot-tying without damaging the sutures.

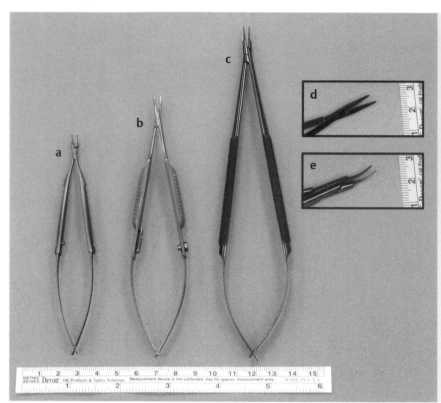

Fig. 2.8 Microsurgical needle holders. Small needle holders are used for superficial bypass procedures, while those with longer handles and curved tips are for anastomoses in a deep surgical field. From left to right, needle holders made of **(a)** titanium (6.6 g) (Charmant, Inc.), **(b)** steel with plastic handle (Aesculap, Inc.), and **(c)** steel with long handle (Mizuho America, Inc.). The tips of the two different microsurgical needle holders in the insets illustrate **(d)** thick straight tips and **(e)** narrow curved tips.

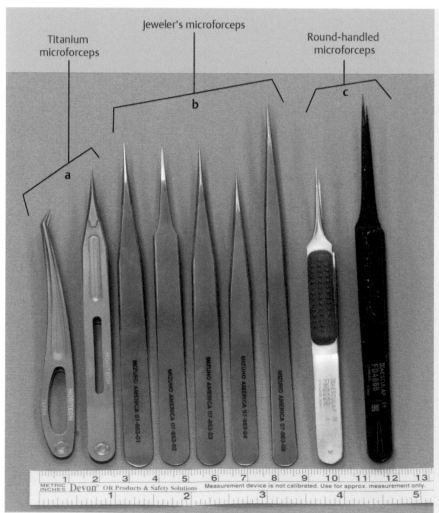

Fig. 2.9 Microforceps. **(a)** Light, titanium nonmagnetic microforceps (Charmant, Inc.). **(b)** Classic set of graduated jeweler's microforceps that differ by the width and length of the tips. From left to right, the first 2 have a strong tip, the third and fourth have a very fine tip, and the fifth has a long tip (Mizuho America, Inc.). **(c)** Microforceps with rounded handles to allow smooth fine rotation movements (Aesculap, Inc.).

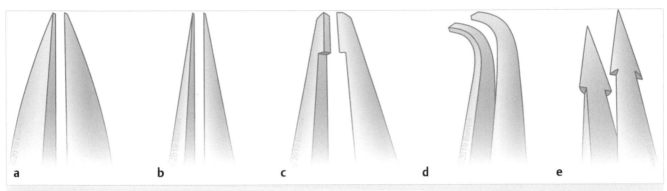

Fig. 2.10 Shape types of microforceps tips. **(a)** Wide, strong tips; **(b)** narrow, fine tips; **(c)** tips with a flat platform (for tying knots); **(d)** curved tips for reaching under a vessel and working in a deep surgical field; and **(e)** cone-shaped plain tips (for vessel dilation).

Vessel Dilators

A vessel dilator is a special type of forceps with cone-shaped plain tips (▸ Fig. 2.10e). This shape facilitates insertion of the instrument into the vessel lumen. The instrument can then be passively opened to delicately widen the vessel orifice. For laboratory training and clinical cases, the vessel dilator is beneficial but not essential.

Scissors

Short straight microscissors are preferable for microsurgery in shallow operative fields, especially for trainees at the beginning of their microsurgical training, because their tips can be manipulated more precisely than the tips of longer instruments (▸ Fig. 2.11). However, in most cases, deep neurosurgical approaches require the use of long microscissors, which can be straight, bayonet-shaped (▸ Fig. 2.12), or single-shafted (▸ Fig. 2.13). Microscissors are the main instruments used for sharp dissection of the arachnoid membrane, and they come with different types of handles and tips. Microscissors are grasped firmly in the hand and then smoothly manipulated by the fingertips to perform delicate and precise movements of the tips. Several types of handle shapes have been designed specifically to improve the handling properties of microscissors. Handles can be flat or rounded, they can have additional bars,[12] and they can have various antiskid surfaces. It is important to use long microscissors for deep work and short microscissors for surface work. Using an instrument with an inappropriate length results in awkward hand positions, fatigue, and a decrease in performance. Microscissors, like microforceps, should be used only for work on delicate tissue. In order to maintain maximal sharpness, the scissors used to incise vessels should be used only for this purpose, with another pair used for microdissection. For skull-base dissections, the microscissors need to be sturdy; they should be made from an extra-hard special alloy and should have a thicker profile. Part of laboratory training involves learning how to choose the right type of microscissors (i.e., by their tips) for the particular surgical situation (▸ Fig. 2.11). For example, using blunt-tipped scissors for vessel dissection can prevent a stabbing injury to an aneurysm or a vessel, yet still easily allow the operator to cut all adhesions captured between the blades. In contrast, the use of sharp-tipped scissors for such a maneuver has a higher risk for unintentional stabbing injury and bleeding.

Microscissors come with various types of tips to accommodate various surgical needs and sharp dissection styles. A key feature is the shape of the tip, which can be straight and flat (▸ Fig. 2.11a), curved (▸ Fig. 2.11d–f), or angled. Straight, flat tips are the most universal and are well-suited for surface dissection. Slightly curved tips are more visible in deep, narrow operative corridors and allow precise control of their position. Flat, slightly angled tips in a crescent shape serve the same purpose and, in addition, allow gentle lifting of the tissue plane during cutting. The tips may also be angled more for dissection at difficult surgical dissection angles (▸ Fig. 2.11g). The tips may be blunt or sharp depending on the dissection needs. The tips also vary by their rigidity, due to the use of different materials and different thicknesses which determine whether the scissors will be used for cutting delicate or tough tissues (microvascular vs. skull base tumor surgery).

Vascular Clips

Microsurgical vascular clips are available in many different types (▸ Fig. 2.14). They can be applied as a single clip or connected in pairs (clip approximators). Among the single clip types, the Mayfield and Kleinert-Kutz types have the advantage of being able to be held by tissue forceps, whereas the Sugita, Yaşargil, and Spetzler types require the appropriate clip applier.[13,14] Clips are made of titanium or steel alloys. Modern clips are compatible with magnetic resonance imaging, but older clips must be checked to determine whether they are ferromagnetic. Clips can be classified by their closing force as temporary (closing force, 50–85 g) and permanent (closing force, 105–185 g), where g equals amount of weight in grams the clips exert.[15] By convention, temporary clips are colored differently than permanent ones, and they are also colored by size to match the appropriate clip applier. Clips are produced in different shapes: straight, curved, and fenestrated, so that single clips or a combination of clips will be suitable for various shapes of aneurysms. Clip approximators may be used for easy approximation of the vessel ends during end-to-end anastomosis. Aproximators can be improvised by taking two Mayfield or

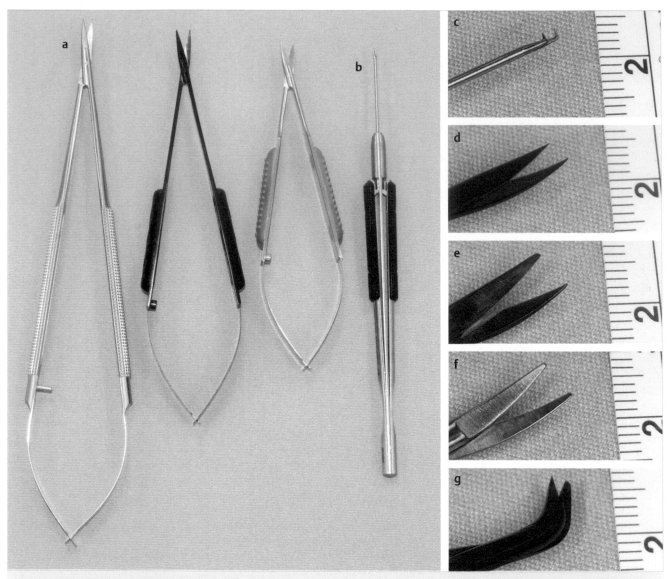

Fig. 2.11 Microscissors are available in various handle lengths, with tips that vary in sharpness, curvature, and rigidity of materials. **(a)** Three different scissors show how any scissors shape can have different lengths for the handle and the shaft to facilitate manipulations performed on the surface and in deep corridors. **(b)** Novel single-shaft instruments minimize obstruction of the view and allow manipulation of the target through a minimally invasive keyhole approach. **(c–g)** Basic shapes of the tips of microscissors include **(c)** arteriotomy microscissors with 60-degree angled tips; **(d)** sharp tips; **(e)** scissors with one sharp tip and one blunt tip for insertion inside the vessel during an arteriotomy; **(f)** blunt tips, which make such instruments safe for blunt dissection; and **(g)** angled tips for deep dissection and for around-the-corner dissection.

Sugita clips and inserting a tightly folded stick of paper into the rings of each clip to hold them parallel.

The application of a temporary or permanent clip is performed according to the aim of the training exercise. The temporary closure of vessels with clips must be done sparingly to avoid damaging the endothelium.

Clip Appliers

The clip applier is used to affix the clip. It allows for the smooth opening and closing of the tips of the clip (▶ Fig. 2.15). Some types of appliers have a handle that allows a 360-degree rotation of the tip (▶ Fig. 2.15a), whereas others have a defined shape and locking mechanism for clip fixation (▶ Fig. 2.15b).

Scalpels

In clinical practice, surgeons use disposable blades to incise the skin and dura (▶ Fig. 2.16). Some neurosurgeons prefer to use special diamond blades for precise microsurgical dissection of the finest structures (▶ Fig. 2.16e, f). However, laboratory costs can be contained by using razor blades and blade holders, which are inexpensive and easily obtained. Care should be exercised to reduce the inherent risk involved in loading the razor blade into the holder.

2.3.5 Bipolar Coagulation Instruments

Bipolar coagulation instruments are not essential for laboratory training because hemostasis can be performed by applying

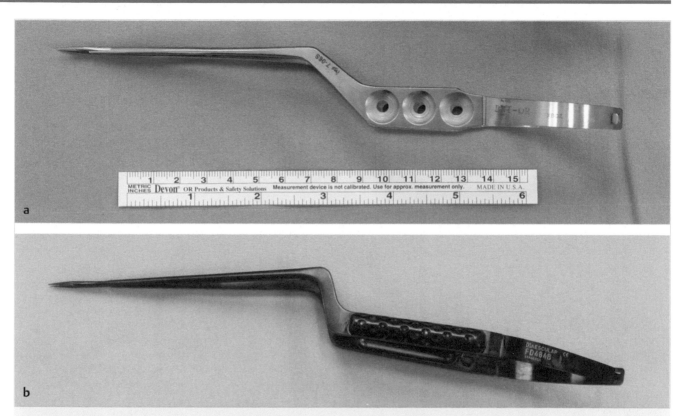

Fig. 2.12 Bayonet-shaped microscissors. **(a)** Yaşargil classic bayoneted microscissors and **(b)** microscissors with an increased bayonet angle designed to reduce interference of the hand with the microscopic view and with a black coating to reduce reflection glint under the microscopic view.

ligatures or pressure with a cotton swab. The use of bipolar forceps for coagulation is often avoided in the microsurgical laboratory because bipolar coagulation can cause vasospasm in small animal vessels, which results in failure of the microanastomosis. However, in clinical microneurosurgery, bipolar forceps are a basic instrument for hemostasis, blunt dissection, and even tissue retraction (▶ Fig. 2.17).[16,17] Good bipolar coagulation is indispensable for creating a clear bloodless operative field, especially for microanastomoses in large animal models and in humans. The main improvements in bipolar forceps in the past decade are in the types of tips being used, for example, gold-plated tips and integrated irrigation to reduce tissue adhesion or ceramic insulated tips to avoid collateral thermal damage.

2.3.6 Retractors

The edges of an operative wound can be retracted either with traditional retractors or with any of several homemade retractors (▶ Fig. 2.18). Custom-made retractors for laboratory bypass on rats can be made of a paper clip attached to a rubber band or of a piece of flexible aluminum wire that can serve as a self-retaining retractor. A sterile retractor can be made from a bent syringe needle attached to a rubber band.

2.3.7 Tissue Irrigators and Solutions for Irrigation

Tissue should be kept moistened not only during real operations but also in laboratory practice sessions. Keeping the tissue

moist minimizes its adhesion to the instruments and sutures. As tissue dries out, it become rigid and fragile, and it loses elasticity. Anastomosis sutures can then easily tear or cut through the dried vessel wall and cause other technical difficulties. Because light from the microscope dries the surface of biological tissue quickly, irrigation with normal saline is necessary, especially when performing microanastomoses. Spray bulbs, syringes with a cut needle or a flexible tip, and wet cotton balls or patties can all be used for irrigation.

In clinical practice, heparinized saline (10–25 units/mL [1,000–2,500 units heparin diluted in 100 mL of saline]) is used for vessel washout and irrigation during anastomosis suturing. The best concentration of heparin for local vessel washout is debatable, with reports documenting a range of concentrations: 10, 100, 250, and 500 units/mL, respectively.[18,19] The anticoagulation property of heparin makes the use of heparinized saline essential when performing anastomoses. In the laboratory, irrigation with heparinized solution is not always necessary (except during wet training) because the aim of the training is not to produce long-term patency but rather to master the necessary technical skills for creating a viable anastomosis. For vasospasm prophylaxis and treatment, peripheral vasodilators may be applied: 15% magnesium sulfate (effective for vessels < 1 mm in diameter) and 1 to 2% lidocaine. The strong vasodilator, papaverine, may also be applied to the vessel externally.

2.3.8 Suction Cannulas

Suction cannulas of different lengths and diameters are essential in the surgical setting, but they are rarely used during

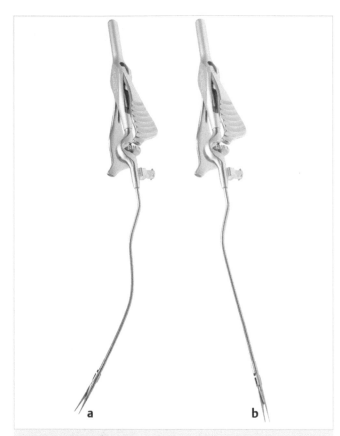

Fig. 2.13 Pliable nitinol microscissors. **(a)** These microscissors can be contoured as needed. **(b)** The microscissors return to their original configuration when heat sterilized. (Images provided courtesy of Peter Lazic, Inc.)

absorbent cotton balls or sticks. In clinical practice, it is more practical to use special absorbent cotton sponges with a ligature, which easily absorb liquid (▶ Fig. 2.20). To protect anatomic structures from damage by suction, the blood or cerebrospinal fluid may be aspirated through the cotton sponge.

2.3.10 Sutures and Needles

The needles and sutures that are used for microsurgery are so thin that they are almost invisible without magnification and easy to lose during surgery. They are the basic materials used for microanastomosis, so trainees must learn the most common sizes and nomenclature (▶ Table 2.2, ▶ Fig. 2.21). Sutures are produced by different companies, and each company uses its own naming system. ▶ Table 2.3 summarizes the nomenclature for several types of sutures and needles produced by Ethicon (Ethicon US, LLC) and S&T (S&T, AG).

Thin, nonabsorbable, monofilament sutures have gained favor in microsurgery. Monofilament sutures do not produce a sawing effect and can easily be pulled through tissue without damaging it. Atraumatic needles with sutures are used to suture veins, arteries, lymphatic vessels, and nerves. Needles with a shape of one-fourth or three-eighths of a circle are more convenient to use in microsurgery. The diameter of both the needle and the suture should correspond to the size of the anastomosis. Usually, the 8–0, 9–0, and 10–0 sutures with taper-point needles and a flattened body are used to anastomose small vessels. The flat profile prevents rotation of the needle in the forceps or needle holder, which can occur with needles with a round profile (▶ Fig. 2.22).

For training purposes, it is reasonable to use cheaper, nonsterile sutures (available from Muranaka Medical Instruments Co. Ltd, Izumi, Osaka, Japan; AROSurgical Instruments, Newport Beach, California, USA, and many other companies that can be found online). Another alternative is to use sutures left over from other operations.

2.3.11 Dyes

Visualization of the thin semitransparent vessel walls can be facilitated with the application of methylene blue, gentian violet, or indigo carmine blue dye (▶ Fig. 2.23). Each anastomosis requires less than a drop of dye, which is carefully applied to the vessel by dipping the microforceps in the dye, like dipping a pen in an inkwell, and then marking the vessel. Microforceps tips are significantly thinner than a surgical marker and allow more accurate and narrow staining. These dyes are benign to the vessel wall, and they significantly increase the visibility of the vessel wall layers.

2.3.12 Background Material

When a vessel is prepared for a bypass, a wedge-shaped background sheet (also known as a rubber dam) can be placed beneath the vessel to improve contrast and to keep the operative field clean and separate from the surrounding brain. These special background strips, which often have a millimeter grid and an antiglare surface, are designed specifically for microsurgical use. For laboratory practice, a piece of latex glove can be used instead.

microsurgical training (▶ Fig. 2.19). Nevertheless, aspiration effectively removes blood and blood clots before they adhere to the endothelium. Suction force is regulated by pressing a finger to the hole in the proximal end of the suction cannula. An aspirator with a linear hole allows accurate regulation of the suction force to avoid damaging tissue or attaching to tissue. This technique helps a surgeon to manipulate the working tip accurately. The suction power can also be changed on the suction device. The intraoperative use of suction cannulas has some nuances. Optimally, suction is used not only for aspiration but also for brain retraction, and to create counterpressure during microsurgical dissection with other instruments. A lighted suction cannula is especially helpful in deep and narrow corridors. The intermittent use of suction to remove cerebrospinal fluid and blood while performing bypasses in a clinical setting is usually cumbersome because it is time consuming and detracts from the actual suturing. Thus, a suction microtube should be placed at the deepest area of the approach near the anastomosis. Doing so allows the operative field to be kept drained and clean even when irrigation is necessary.

2.3.9 Sponges and Gauze

Sponges or small cotton pellets are used to drain the operative field to remove liquid or blood and to moisten and protect anatomic structures. In the laboratory, it is easy to use cosmetic

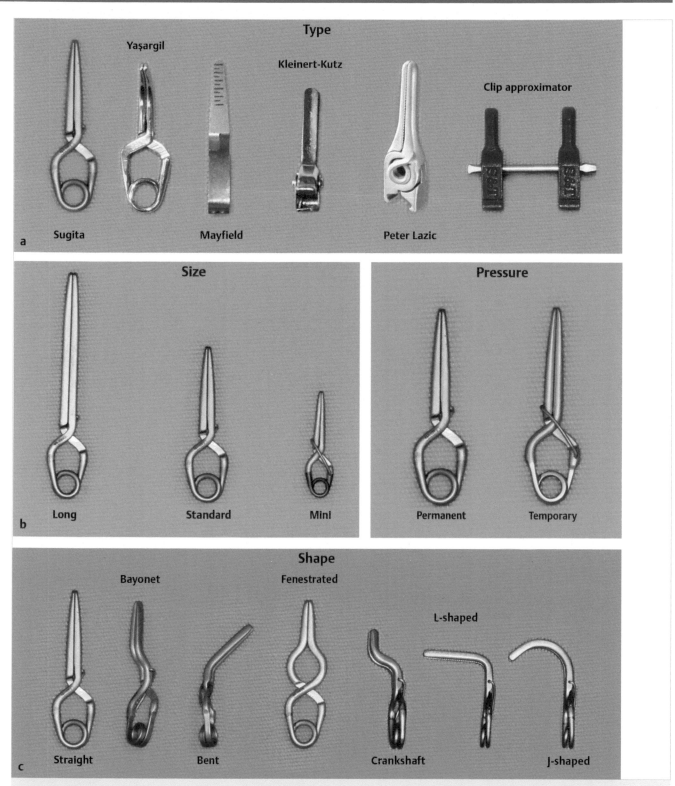

Fig. 2.14 Neurosurgical vascular clips. Clips can be classified by type, size, closing pressure, and shape. **(a)** The most common types of clips are the spirally bent Sugita and Yaşargil clips. Less commonly used are the flat Mayfield clip with a single bend and the spring-loaded Kleinert-Kutz clip. The Peter Lazic (Peter Lazic, GmbH) clip has a reversed opening mechanism to minimize the needle holder's obstruction of the view of the surgical field. An approximator is used to bring two ends of the vessel together for anastomosis. **(b)** Clip sizes range from miniature to long, and the degree of pressure they apply can be temporary or permanent. **(c)** The various clip shapes include straight, bayoneted, bent, fenestrated, crankshaft, L-shaped, and J-shaped. (Fig. 2.14a, Peter Lazic clip provided courtesy of Peter Lazic, Inc.)

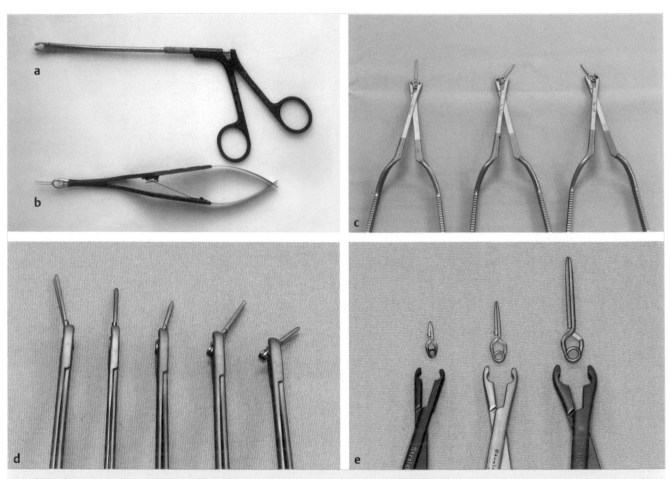

Fig. 2.15 Clip appliers. The main types of clip appliers are **(a)** the single shaft clip applier with a 360-degree rotation for narrow approaches (Aesculap, Inc.) and **(b)** the standard bayonet-shaped clip applier with a locking mechanism (Aesculap, Inc.). **(c, d)** Clip appliers differ by the direction in which the clip is held and moved, either **(c)** horizontal or **(d)** vertical, and **(e)** by the size of clip they can hold.

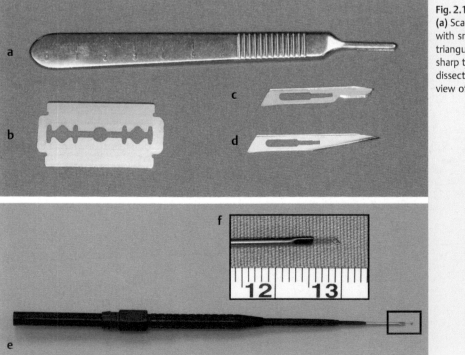

Fig. 2.16 Scalpel handle and surgical blades. **(a)** Scalpel handle no. 3; **(b)** razor blade; **(c)** blade with small curved cutting edge (no. 15); **(d)** triangular blade with straight cutting edge and sharp tip (no. 11); and **(e)** diamond blade for fine dissection with **(f)** inset demonstrating magnified view of small diamond tip of blade.

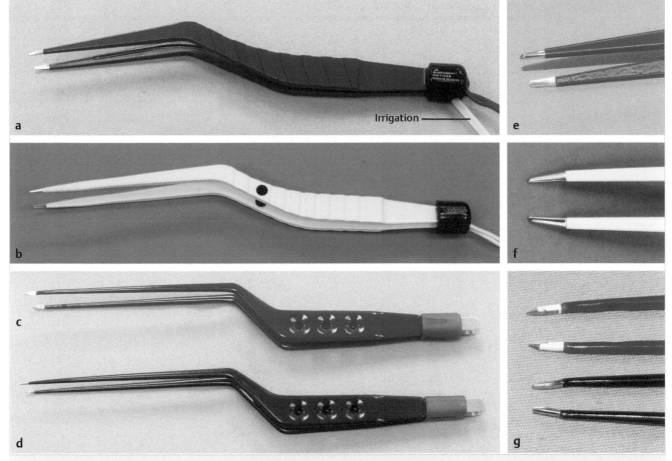

Fig. 2.17 Bayonet-shaped bipolar forceps with working shafts of various lengths are used in neurosurgery. Reusable and disposable bipolar forceps are available with **(a, b)** an increased angle for more comfortable handling as well as **(c, d)** the classic bayonet shape. **(e–g)** The best bipolar forceps are those with nonstick tips. **(e, f)** Tips made of a high heat-conducting material, such as silver, will cool down between applications of coagulation. Tips are made in full metal (**g**, *lower forceps*) or are ceramic covered (**g**, *upper forceps*) to protect surrounding tissues from heat damage. More recent developments in the tips of bipolar forceps include built-in irrigation to further decrease tissue adherence (*as shown in* **a**). (Instruments provided by Kogent Surgical [**a, b**] and Aesculap, Inc. [**c, d**].)

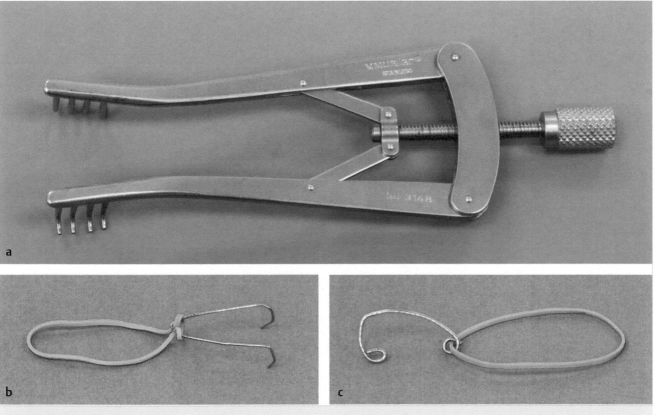

Fig. 2.18 Retractors for laboratory practice. **(a)** Traditional self-retaining serrated retractor. **(b, c)** Custom retractors made from a paper clip and a rubber band.

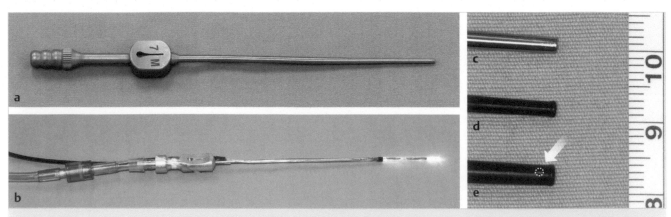

Fig. 2.19 Suction cannulas. **(a)** Suction cannulas consist of a rigid or malleable tube and a handle with a teardrop-shaped hole to control the force of the suction. **(b)** Suction devices with lighted tips are designed for deep keyhole approaches. **(c–e)** In contrast to the standard end of a surgical aspirator **(c)**, the blunt ball-shaped atraumatic tip of the suction cannula **(d, e)** avoids trauma to delicate tissues and allows the use of the suction device as a dissector. A small hole **(e,** *arrow and dotted circle*) near the tip of the cannula facilitates removal of blood and cerebrospinal fluid and avoids damage from excess suction while preventing tissue from clinging to the cannula.

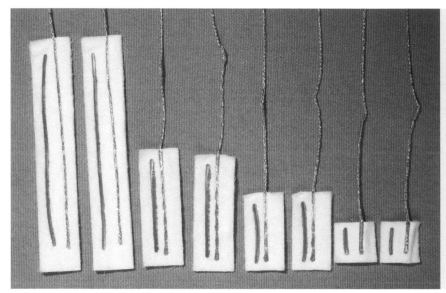

Fig. 2.20 Cottonoid. A wide range of sizes of absorbent cotton sponges is essential in neurosurgery. Cottonoids should be marked in a manner that allows them to be seen on radiographs (shown as a *blue stripe* on these cottonoids), and they should have an attached suture for easy atraumatic removal.

Table 2.2 Size of suture filaments

USP designation	EP designation (i.e., metric size)	Diameter, mm	
		Minimum	Maximum
12–0	0.01	0.001	0.009
11–0	0.1	0.010	0.019
10–0	0.2	0.020	0.029
9–0	0.3	0.030	0.039
8–0	0.4	0.040	0.049

Abbreviations: EP, European Pharmacopoeia; USP, United States Pharmacopeia.

Table 2.3 Nomenclature of sutures and needles

Company	Name	Explanation
Ethicon US, LLC	BV 75–3 BVH 100–3 ST 75–4	BV = blood vessel 75 = Needle diameter, μm 3 = chord length, mm H = half-circle ST = straight needle
S&T, AG	7V43	7 = needle diameter of 70 μm V = vascular 4 = chord length, mm 3 = 3/8 of circle

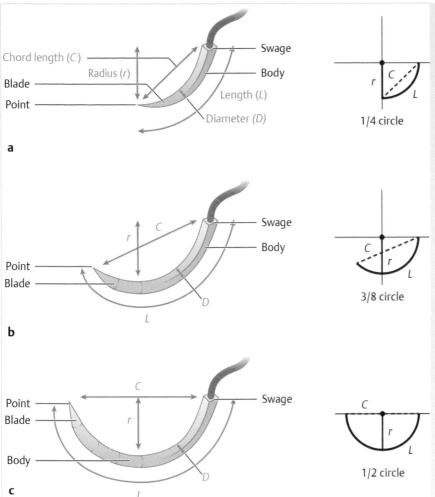

Chord length (C)
Radius (r)
Blade
Point
Swage
Body
Length (L)
Diameter (D)

a

r C
L
1/4 circle

Fig. 2.21 Nomenclature of surgical needles. Illustration shows curved needles that are **(a)** one-quarter circle, **(b)** three-eighths circle, and **(c)** one-half circle. The characteristics of a needle are described using the following terms: chord length (C), radius (r), length (L), diameter (D), blade, point, body, and swage. The chord length is the straight distance from the swage end to the tip; the radius is the radius of the extrapolated full circle.

r C
Swage
Body
Point
Blade
D
L

b

C
r
L
3/8 circle

C
r
Point
Blade
Body
D
L
Swage

c

C
r
L
1/2 circle

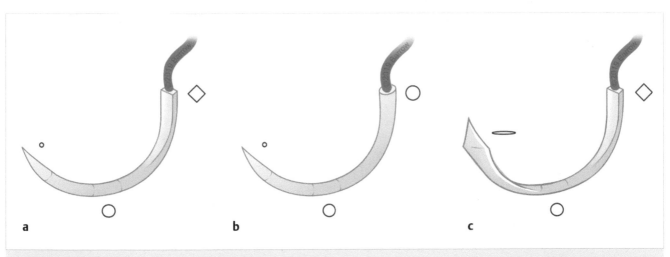

a   **b**   **c**

Fig. 2.22 Types of surgical needles. **(a)** Tapered point needle with round section on tip and flattened section on body (for vascular microanastomosis in humans); **(b)** needle with round section along its full length (for training); and **(c)** needle with lancet tip (for ophthalmology).

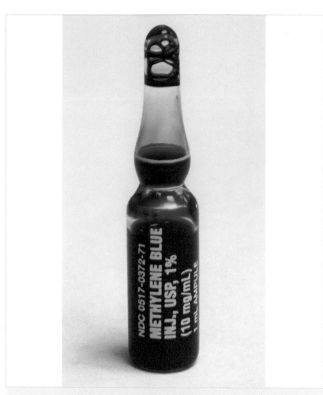

Fig. 2.23 Methylene blue, 1% solution, may be used to stain the walls of small vessels during bypass to improve visualization of the layers and edges.

2.3.13 High-Speed Drills

Learning how to use a high-speed drill to develop good bone dissection skills will ultimately enable the trainee to perform successful craniotomies and to create pathways for vascular bypasses with minimal trauma and fewer drill-related complications. Drill bits come in different shapes and sizes for use not only for the craniotomy but also for dissection and decompression of nerves and vessels within bony canals. In the training laboratory, drilling skills can be perfected with practice on large animal models (e.g., bovine scapula and skull and sheep spine) and during cadaveric dissections. Delicate bone work with the microsurgical drill can be practiced on the shells of raw chicken eggs and on animal bones (▶ Fig. 2.24). A thorough explanation of bone dissection can be found in a temporal bone dissection guide.[20] The basic principles are: irrigate copiously and constantly during drilling to remove debris and prevent heat-induced injury; use diamond bits for delicate and slowly performed dissection; use fluted drill bits for fast bone removal; and avoid the use of gauze while drilling.

2.4 Devices for Simulation of a Deep Operative Field

Many different support stands can be used to simulate the approach to a deep operative field (▶ Fig. 2.25). The simplest of these can be made by the trainees themselves simply by cutting a hole in a cardboard or plastic carton or box or by cutting a hole in an inverted plastic bowl. Plastic building bricks (Lego, The Lego Group) can also be stacked to create a stand with adjustable height.

2.5 Costs of Instruments and Alternatives to Purchasing

When faced with insufficient economic resources to purchase expensive microsurgical instruments, it is wise to check with the operating room manager as to whether satisfactory instruments that are being discarded after procedures may be sent to the laboratory instead. Training grants from neurosurgery equipment companies may also provide some instruments to the laboratory. In addition, many equipment companies have second- or third-order lines of instruments that are satisfactory for use in the training setting but are not as high quality as more expensive lines for human use. Sometimes when a hospital purchases instruments for use in the operating room, the equipment company will agree to donate lower-grade instruments for the training laboratory. Alternatively, lower-cost jeweler's and veterinary instruments or used neurosurgery instruments are frequently available in the open market and can be purchased over the Internet (▶ Table 2.4). These lower-quality instruments are appropriate for initial laboratory practice, but the improved microsurgical performance with high-quality microsurgical instruments should serve as a motivation to obtain them.

2.6 Conclusion

In conclusion, the trainee should acquire a personalized set of microsurgical instruments based on their availability, the goals of training, and the training model. ▶ Fig. 2.26 displays the minimal set required for microsurgical training. Regardless of whether the training laboratory facilities and equipment are simply the bare essentials or state of the art, it is the motivation and dedication of the trainee that enables them to become a neurosurgeon who is skilled in microsurgical techniques. A compelling desire to learn and dedicated and regular practice sessions in even the most basically outfitted laboratory are even more important than access to the finest tools available.

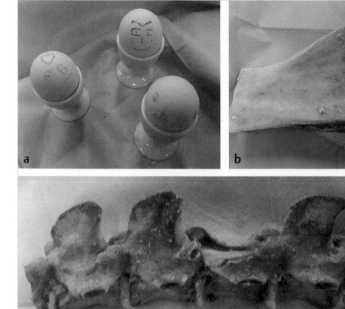

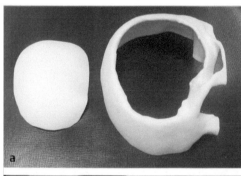

Fig. 2.24 Laboratory training exercises use a high-speed drill and various materials to develop delicate drilling skills. **(a)** Drilling performed on an uncooked egg without perforating the membrane. **(b)** Drilling practiced on a bovine scapula. **(c)** A laminectomy and foraminotomies performed on a sheep spine.

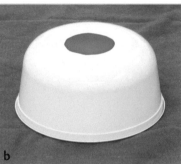

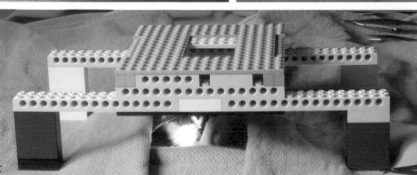

Fig. 2.25 Support stands for simulation of a deep operative field. **(a)** A three-dimensional printed model of a skull with a craniotomy. **(b)** A deep-sided, flat-bottomed bowl with a center-cut hole turned upside down. **(c)** A stand for arm support and depth simulation made from plastic toy building bricks (Lego, The Lego Group).

Table 2.4 Average cost of minimal microsurgical bypass training tools and equipment

Item	No. needed	Low-cost solution (various online sources)			High-grade solution		
		Description	Average cost	Total	Description	Average cost	Total cost
Dissection microscope	1	Stereomicroscope, laboratory grade with fixed head	$800	$800	Stereomicroscope with changeable magnification and movable head (surgical grade)	$10,000–$500,000	Wide range[a]
Forceps (jeweler's)	2	Training grade	$10	$20	Microsurgical high-quality grade	$500	$1,000
Microsurgical needle holder	1	Training grade	$20	$20	Microsurgical high-quality grade	$1,000	$1,000
Yaşargil bayoneted microscissors	1	Training grade	$60	$60	Microneurosurgical high-quality grade	$1,000	$1,000
Silicone tube (1–2 mm diameter)	1	Technical or food grade	$2	$2	Polyvinyl alcohol hydrogel microvessels	$100	$100
10–0 or 9–0 sutures	2	Training grade, nonsterile	$3	$6	Microvascular grade	$330	$660
Microvascular clips	2	Schwartz type	$20	$40	Microsurgical aneurysm clips or surgical grade approximator	$200	$400
Clip applier	1	Optional	$200[a]	$200 [a]	Neurosurgical grade	$500	$500
Total cost				**$948**			**$4,660 +**

[a]The cost is not included in the calculation of the total cost.
Source: Adapted from Belykh et al.[5]

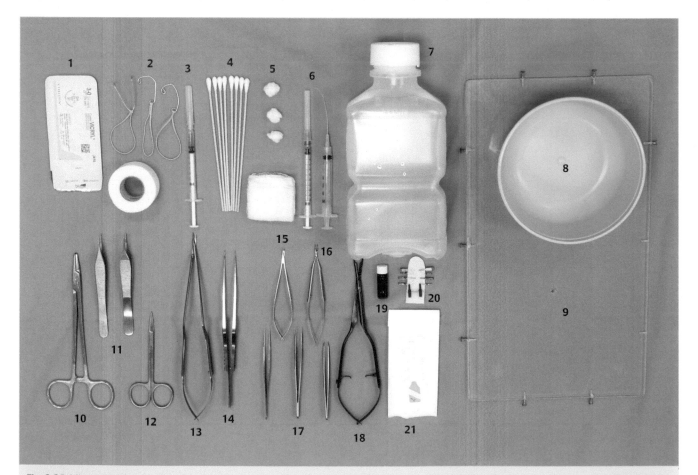

Fig. 2.26 Microsurgical instruments for laboratory training. At a minimum, laboratory training requires the following set of instruments: (1) Sutures for retraction, vessel ligation, and closure; (2) retractors (at least two); (3) anesthetic; (4, 5) sponges or cotton balls or swabs (6) syringes with thin needles; (7) heparin sodium (flushing solution); (8) bowl for washing solution; (9) small operating board for animal fixation; (10) macroneedle holder (for skin closure); (11) surgical forceps (for macrosurgical steps); (12) eye scissors (for macrosurgical steps); (13) long microscissors (for deep-field exercises); (14) long microforceps (for deep-field exercises); (15) short microscissors; (16) microsurgical needle holders; (17) microforceps (two or three); (18) microsurgical clip applicator; (19) dye (methylene blue); (20) microsurgical or aneurysm clips and a rubber dam (e.g., from a glove); and (21) 8–0, 9–0, or 10–0 sutures (for microanastomosis).

References

[1] Martins PN, Montero EF. Organization of a microsurgery laboratory. Acta Cir Bras; 21(3):187–189

[2] Yaşargil MG. From the microsurgical laboratory to the operating theatre. Acta Neurochir (Wien); 147(5):465–468

[3] Izci Y, Timurkaynak E. A short history of the microsurgery training and research laboratory at Gulhane Military Medical Academy. Turk Neurosurg; 20(2):269–273

[4] Green CJ. Organisation of a microsurgical laboratory. Br J Plast Surg; 43(6):641–644

[5] Belykh E, Byvaltsev V. Off-the-job microsurgical training on dry models: Siberian experience. World Neurosurg; 82(1–2):20–24

[6] Aoun SG, El Ahmadieh TY, El Tecle NE, et al. A pilot study to assess the construct and face validity of the Northwestern Objective Microanastomosis Assessment Tool. J Neurosurg; 123(1):103–109

[7] Omahen DA. The 10,000-hour rule and residency training. CMAJ; 180(12):1272

[8] Pitskhelauri DI, Konovalov AN, Shekutev GA, et al. A novel device for hands-free positioning and adjustment of the surgical microscope. J Neurosurg; 121(1):161–164

[9] Mamelak AN, Nobuto T, Berci G. Initial clinical experience with a high-definition exoscope system for microneurosurgery. Neurosurgery; 67(2):476–483

[10] Birch K, Drazin D, Black KL, Williams J, Berci G, Mamelak AN. Clinical experience with a high definition exoscope system for surgery of pineal region lesions. J Clin Neurosci; 21(7):1245–1249

[11] O'Brien MC, Morrison WA. Micro-instrumentation and microsurgery Reconstructive Microsurgery. 2nd ed. Edinburgh: Churchill Livingstone; 1987

[12] Matsumura N. A new bayonet spring microsurgical instrument handle with a bar for microneurosurgery. Surg Neurol Int; 3:152

[13] Fox JL. Vascular clips for the microsurgical treatment of stroke. Stroke; 7(5):489–500

[14] Louw DF, Asfora WT, Sutherland GR. A brief history of aneurysm clips. Neurosurg Focus; 11(2):E4

[15] Dujovny M, Kossovsky N, Laha RK, Leff L, Wackenhut N, Perlin A. Temporary microvascular clips. Neurosurgery; 5(4):456–463

[16] Spetzler RF, Sanai N. The quiet revolution: retractorless surgery for complex vascular and skull base lesions. J Neurosurg; 116(2):291–300

[17] Chen RK, Than KD, Wang AC, Park P, Shih AJ. Comparison of thermal coagulation profiles for bipolar forceps with different cooling mechanisms in a porcine model of spinal surgery. Surg Neurol Int; 4:113

[18] Cox GW, Runnels S, Hsu HS, Das SK. A comparison of heparinised saline irrigation solutions in a model of microvascular thrombosis. Br J Plast Surg; 45(5):345–348

[19] O'Shaughessy M. Heparinised saline solutions. Br J Plast Surg; 46(3):268

[20] Francis HF, Niparko JK. Temporal Bone Dissection Guide. 2nd ed. New York, NY: Thieme; 2016

3 Day 2: Dry-Laboratory Microsurgical Training: Techniques and Manual Skills

Evgenii Belykh and Nikolay Martirosyan

Abstract

Microvascular operations should not be performed on patients until after the surgeon has undergone an extensive period of laboratory training. In this chapter, we describe basic practical aspects of microneurosurgical techniques that can be mastered during dry microsurgical training. We describe instrument-holding techniques, knot-tying techniques, various anastomosis techniques, and specific microsurgical exercises that are meant to guide the development of tremor control, mindfulness, exact manipulating patterns, and fast knot tying.

Keywords: counter-press method, dry microsurgical training, end-to-end anastomosis, end-to-side anastomosis, instrument-holding techniques, microsurgical knot-tying techniques, side-to-side anastomosis, snowflake exercise, tremor control

3.1 Techniques and Manual Skills

The mastery of microsurgical techniques requires time, special physical skills, motivation, patience, devotion, and a specially equipped workplace. Even experienced surgeons cannot perform microsurgical operations without specialized preparatory training.

Speed—not haste—must be part of the skill set of the neurosurgeon, because the duration of the surgical intervention necessary to create anastomoses is significant: the extent of ischemic and reperfusion injuries increases with the passage of time. Therefore, a neurosurgeon must not only have a suitable skill level in terms of precision and accuracy but also possess and cultivate operative speed. Idiosyncrasies such as impatience, insufficient coordination of movements, and tremor weigh heavily on the neurosurgeon's ability to perform microneurosurgery. Laboratory training can be used to correct these problems through practice and adaptation or, in some cases, by convincing a trainee that a clinical focus on the practice of microsurgery is not the best career choice.

Furthermore, the work of the neurosurgeon must combine laboratory exercises with clinical practice to perfect practical skills and to learn new technologies. This chapter covers the fundamental background information that is necessary to master microsurgical techniques effectively and quickly.

Sidebar

- The tips and tenets described in this chapter are to be used throughout the rest of the training.
- Dry training and a warm-up exercise set, as described below, are to be used repetitively and continuously in the resident's or doctor's office to save on training time in the laboratory.

3.2 Mental Concentration

Microsurgical training sessions should have scheduled breaks. Trainees should not overwork during this training, because being tired significantly decreases the educational value of the training, and it becomes a waste of time. If you feel tired after 1 or 2 hours of training, you should get up and walk away from the table for a few minutes to cleanse your mind and reduce muscle fatigue. You should return to practice only when you feel refreshed and can approach the exercises with a positive attitude toward mastering the skills.

Since the microsurgical world represents a completely different experience for even the experienced surgeon, numerous difficulties and obstacles are inevitable during training. Thus, you should learn how to avoid feeling frustrated. Difficulties with the exercises often lead to frustration and despair. In a desperate state, problems only get worse: sutures become tangled, the needle bends, and the tissue ruptures. By stopping and thinking about what creates such difficulties, you can identify the reason for your frustration, which may be a very simple obstacle, such as bad hand position, bad hemostasis, or maladjustment of the microscope. Eventually, the surgeon should develop a mental checklist of preparatory actions that can be effectively deployed during pauses taken to think through each difficulty and the reasons for it.

A quiet atmosphere in the operating room, which promotes tranquility and emotional stability in the operating surgeon are also important requirements for microneurosurgery. Leading neurosurgeons of the United States, Japan, and Europe recommend playing quiet classical music or having complete silence in the operating room.

3.3 Position of the Operator

Special attention should be paid to the position and height of the operating table and chair, the position of the operative microscope, the location of the necessary equipment and tools, and the choice of the method for hemostasis. The microsurgical training (the same as the microsurgical stage of the operation) is performed in the sitting position, with the forearms, wrists, and fingers on elbow rests or on the table in a physiologically natural position. Surgeons sometimes pride themselves on their ability to battle against fatigue and discomfort, but during microsurgery is not the time to exercise this fortitude, as it will be needed for the work itself. Comfort is not a luxury during microneurosurgery but instead is an absolute requirement. A comfortable position is defined as a position with the minimum number of muscles working. The arms must be in a relaxed position that can be maintained as long as necessary. The stance of the surgeon should be completely comfortable, without any tension. The back and neck should be straight, the forearms should be placed horizontally, and the feet should be resting comfortably on the floor or on a footrest; this position creates three points of support, which significantly decreases the work of back muscles that support stability. This position may require small but important adjustments of the surgical chair or table, which some nurses may find picky. This attitude should not deter the resident or young neurosurgeon, because a comfortable position is one of the essential components for success. The need for a more comfortable position should not arise during the operation or training, but instead should be foreseen and obtained as an essential preparatory step. Shoulders, forearms, and hands must be relaxed. This is only possible when the center of gravity of the forearm is located on the table. We maintain that a microneurosurgical operation cannot be performed optimally without elbow rests. Nevertheless, some well-known neurosurgeons (e.g., Dr. Juha Hernesniemi [Helsinki University Hospital, Helsinki, Finland] and Dr. Alexander Konovalov [Burdenko Neurosurgical Institute, Moscow, Russia]) perform the microsurgical stages of the operation without elbow rests. If the use of elbow rests is impossible, the forearms may be stabilized with the help of a standing armrest or a wrist rest affixed to the head holder.

To avoid eye fatigue caused by the changes in focal distance, you should avoid taking your eyes off the microscope oculars. Microneurosurgeons should have good vision and a good line of sight, and they should be able to use instruments dexterously with both hands. Neurosurgeons who usually wear eyeglasses should also wear them while working with the microscope.

3.4 Managing Tremor

Under normal circumstances, everyone has some degree of tremor. Whether the use of tobacco or alcohol increases tremor in surgeons performing microsurgery has not been confirmed, but their use should be discouraged.[1] Caffeinated coffee is known to affect tremor but only when consumed in larger quantities than is normal for the individual, with no effects on tremor by a habitual coffee drinker when consumption is moderate. Hard manual exercises may affect tremor by increasing resting muscular tone, so heavy muscular strengthening workouts should be avoided for at least 1 day before surgery. Annoyance is another factor that may increase the likelihood of tremor. Neurosurgeons should therefore learn how to avoid becoming irritated. Having a mental checklist, knowing what to prepare, and determining how to deal with difficulties are key to achieving calmness and reducing annoyance.

In some instances, beta-blockers are used to decrease both anxiety and tremor in the arms. Beta-blockers are also used for the same purpose by marksmen. (Beta blockers are on the World Anti-Doping Agency's list of prohibited substances for archery, shooting, and other sports.[2]) Several studies[3,4,5] that have shown a decrease in tremor with beta-blockers (propranolol 10–40 mg) found no effect on the quality of the anastomosis or improvement in the overall surgical results. We believe that the use of beta-blockers is acceptable if it really helps a trainee but that the primary victory over tremor emanates from other important factors. The first key factor is a comfortable position that decreases stiffness and fatigue. A comfortable position helps to fight essential tremor, which is found in everyone to some degree and which increases with exhaustion. Short intervals of rest can also be useful in minimizing essential tremor. Another key factor is appropriate hand position with the entire forearm and wrist resting on the table surface (or support stand) to minimize muscle strain (▶ Fig. 3.1). All these factors (i.e., the skill in manipulating the instruments, the inner calmness, and the ability to suppress nervousness) can be learned through frequent training.

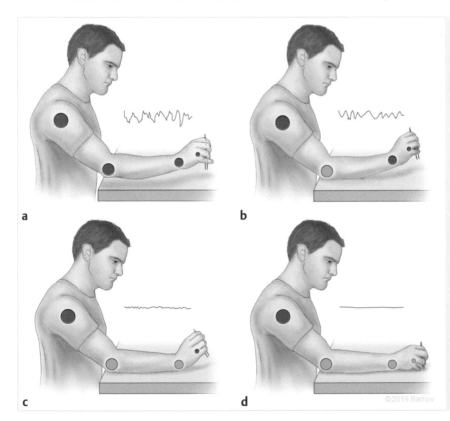

Fig. 3.1 Illustration depicting the importance of hand position to decrease tremor at the tip of the working instrument. **(a)** When there is no arm contact with the table surface, the instrument picks up large oscillations from the whole trunk, the middle-amplitude tremor from the arm, and low-amplitude tremor from the forearm muscles. **(b)** The elbow is stabilized: the high-amplitude tremor from the body disappears, but the tension from the shoulder and forearm muscles still produces tremor. **(c)** When the hand is supported, the low-amplitude tremor is still present due to the work of extensor and abductor muscles in the forearm. **(d)** When the fourth and fifth fingers rest on the surface, the forearm muscles are more relaxed, and there is almost no tremor.

©2019 Barrow

3.5 Techniques for Holding Microsurgical Instruments

The trainee must study how to hold and manipulate different microsurgical instruments. Holding instruments as one holds a pen or chopsticks is considered optimal. The finger pads must be placed one-third of the way from the tip of the instrument. Manipulating the shaft of the instrument as one does chopsticks is the key movement for the use of microsurgery instruments (▶ Fig. 3.2). One shaft of the microsurgery instrument, as in using chopsticks, is held with three bearing points (two fingers and the cusp of the hand), which keeps it well-fixed. The other shaft of the instrument is held and moved with the other fingers. This technique allows full control of the movement of the instrument's tips.

The spring tension of the springy instruments, such as forceps, scissors, and needle holders, is also important. If the tension is too weak, keeping the instrument stable will be difficult. If the tension is too strong, the sensitivity and the ability to perform microscopic movements will erode, leading to tiredness and tremor.

To test for the right tension and to select the appropriate instrument, one should hold the springy instrument and close it partially. Then, fixed in this position, one should rotate the hand. If the tips of the instrument cannot be easily maintained at a fixed distance, the tension is inappropriate. Obtaining the appropriate tension is difficult at first and requires both practice in general and familiarity with the specific instrument being used. The degree of hand fatigue after a period of long training is the best indicator of proper tension. The longer a surgeon can hold the instrument partially closed, the longer he or she will be able to use the instrument during the operation without fatigue compromising microsurgical effectiveness.

3.5.1 Techniques for Holding Short Microforceps

"Reverse holding" technique (▶ Fig. 3.3a): In the reverse holding technique, one arm of the forceps is held in a fixed position by the pads of the forefinger and middle finger. The instrument is directed toward the surgeon, its proximal part against the forefinger. The thumb is opposed to the middle and index fingers and presses down on the second arm of the instrument.

"Index push" technique (▶ Fig. 3.3b): In the index push technique, the lower arm of the instrument is held in a fixed position by the pads of the thumb and middle finger. The instrument is directed away from the surgeon, and the tips are placed one over the other. The proximal part is rested on the first dorsal interosseous muscle near the joint at the base of the forefinger. The index finger presses down on the second arm.

"Traditional" technique (▶ Fig. 3.3c): In the traditional technique, one arm of the instrument is held in a fixed position by the

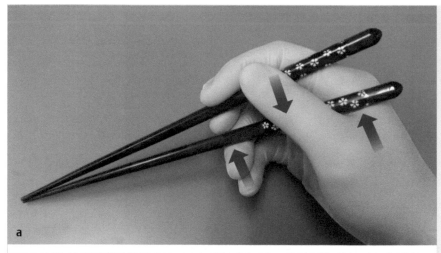

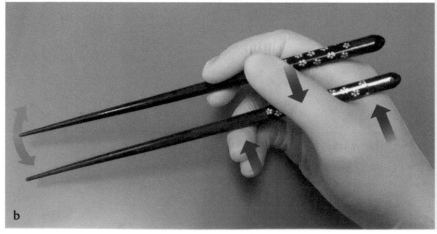

Fig. 3.2 Exercise with chopsticks (simulation of holding microscissors or microforceps). **(a)** One chopstick is fixed (*lower chopstick*). **(b)** Grasping and holding is performed by movement of the other chopstick (*upper chopstick*). *Purple arrows* indicate the points of contact between the hand and instrument; *green arrows* indicate the resulting motion.

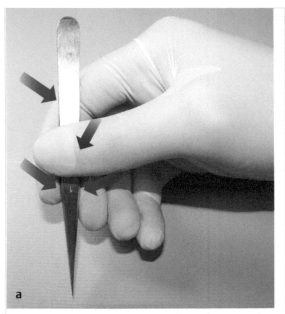
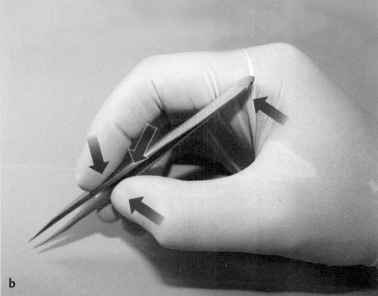
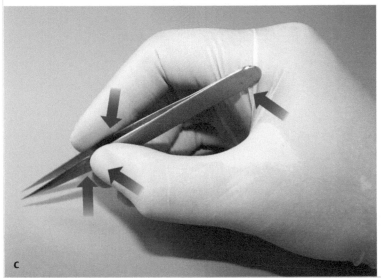
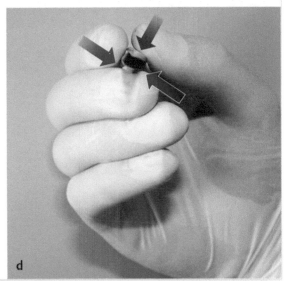

Fig. 3.3 Techniques for holding short microforceps. **(a)** "Reverse holding" technique (Video 3.1). **(b)** "Index push" technique (Video 3.2). **(c)** "Traditional" technique (Video 3.3). **(d)** A reverse view showing the traditional technique for holding the instrument. *Purple arrows* indicate the points of contact between the hand and instrument; *pink arrows* indicate motion needed to close instrument.

pads of the index and middle fingers. The proximal part rests near the joint at the base of the forefinger. The thumb is opposed to the index and middle fingers, so that a triangular shape can be seen from the top of the instrument (▶ Fig. 3.3d). Grasping occurs by pressing down with the thumb. Working in this position for an extended period of time can increase essential tremor in the thumb. The trick for reducing this tremor is to position the thumb so that its tip touches and rests on the index finger, while instrument closure is made by further squeezing these three fingers.

3.5.2 Techniques for Holding Short Straight Microscissors

"Reverse holding" technique (▶ Fig. 3.4a): In the reverse holding technique, the lower shaft is held in a fixed position by the pads

of the index and middle fingers. The instrument is directed back toward the surgeon, its proximal part lying along the distal half of the index finger. The thumb is opposed to the middle and index fingers, and the thumb presses down on the second shaft of the instrument. This technique allows the right-handed surgeon to dissect in a right-to-left direction and toward the surgeon.

"Index push" technique (▶ Fig. 3.4b): In the index push technique, one shaft of the instrument is held in a fixed position by the pads of the thumb and middle finger and stabilized along its length by the side of the forefinger base joint. The microscissors are directed straight forward or to the side from oneself while the jaws of the scissors are oriented vertically one over the other. The forefinger presses down on the second shaft to effect closure. This technique allows you to perform right-handed dissection away from yourself in a wide range toward the left.

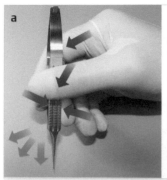
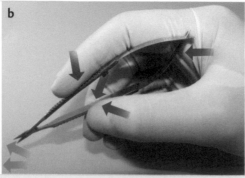
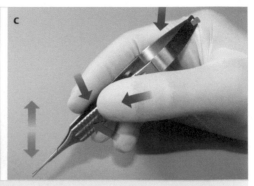

Fig. 3.4 Techniques for holding short straight microscissors (Video 3.4). **(a)** "Reverse holding" technique (Video 3.5). **(b)** "Index push" technique (Video 3.6). **(c)** "Traditional" technique (Video 3.7). *Purple arrows* indicate points of contact to hold the stable shaft of the instrument, *pink arrows* indicate the motion needed to move the movable shaft of the instrument, and *green arrows* indicate directions for cutting and sharp dissection.

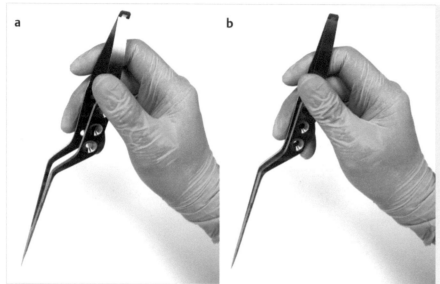

Fig. 3.5 "Traditional" technique for holding long bayonet microscissors. The traditional technique is best for dissection from side to side (Video 3.8). **(a)** The fingertips of the index, middle, and ring fingers hold one shaft of the instrument, while the thumb is positioned on the other side. **(b)** The scissors are closed by simultaneous movement of both halves of the instrument toward each other. The fingers do not obstruct the microscopic view because of the bayonet shape of the instrument shaft.

"Traditional" technique (▶ Fig. 3.4c): In the traditional technique, one shaft of the instrument is held in a fixed position by the pads and length of the forefinger and middle fingers. The other shaft is situated on the main pad of the phalangeal part of the thumb, and movement of this shaft is effected by opposing pressure of the thumb.

3.5.3 Techniques for Holding Long Bayonet Microscissors

Most neurosurgical scissors have a bayonet shape and are considered as the primary tool for sharp arachnoid dissection in cerebrovascular surgery. Rigid tremor-free grasping of the bayonet scissors and delicate dissection are possible using the traditional holding technique. However, familiarity with other holding techniques may not only improve maneuverability and increase confidence in performing dissection from different positions and approaches but also provide the advantage of incorporating smooth instrument tip movements in the various planes and directions.[6] ▶ Fig. 3.5, ▶ Fig. 3.6, ▶ Fig. 3.7, ▶ Fig. 3.8

illustrate different holding techniques for long microscissors (traditional, reverse holding, index push, and "chopsticks" holding techniques). The traditional way of holding bayonet microscissors may require wrist bending in several positions, which is not physiologically optimal, especially when working on the surface of the brain. A set of bayoneted microscissors of varying blade length is usually used during surgery in order to retain proper handling and measurability. Instruments are changed to the longer blades as the dissection progresses deeper.

3.5.4 Stable Hand Positioning

To stabilize the instrument position and to decrease hand tension and fatigue, you can use hand contact techniques: one or more fingers carry out the function of support (▶ Fig. 3.9). This technique is helpful for laboratory use but is not always acceptable under operating conditions. Depending on the situation, a light touch against the patient may be maintained by the hypothenar eminence or the tips of the fingers to assist in stability.

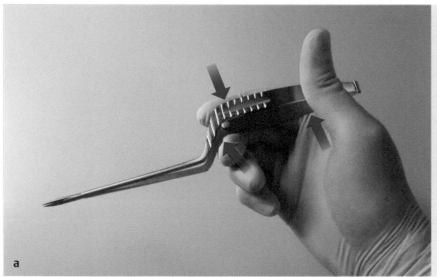

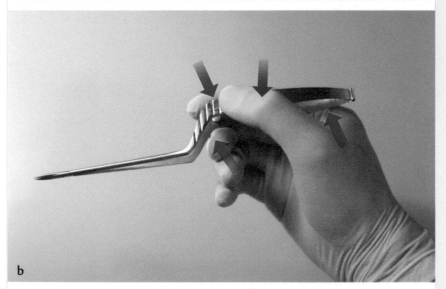

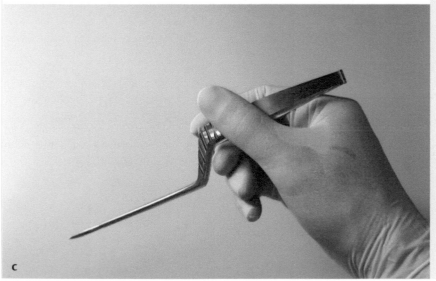

Fig. 3.6 "Reverse holding" (also known as the Japanese style) technique for holding long bayonet microscissors. The reverse holding technique is best for dissection toward yourself (Video 3.9). **(a)** The middle finger is bent in the shape of the bayonet bend of the microscissors. The lower shaft of the instrument is held below with the help of the middle finger. This shaft is held in a fixed position on top by the forefinger so that it is rigidly secured between the index and middle fingers. **(b)** The thumb holds the upper shaft from the top. The upper shaft of the instrument is moved by pressing down with the thumb. **(c)** This technique allows dissection from right to left and toward yourself. *Purple arrows* indicate points of contact between the hand and the stable shaft of the instrument; *pink arrows* indicate the motion needed to move the movable shaft of the instrument.

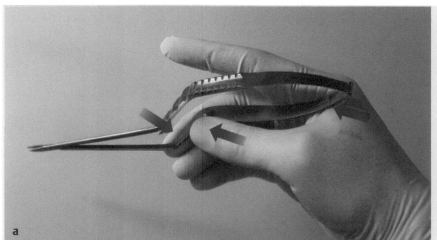

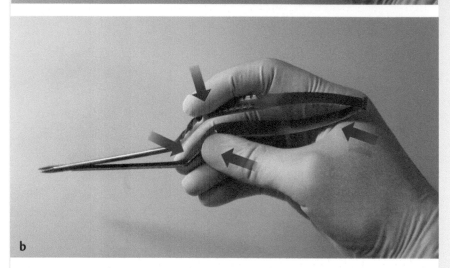

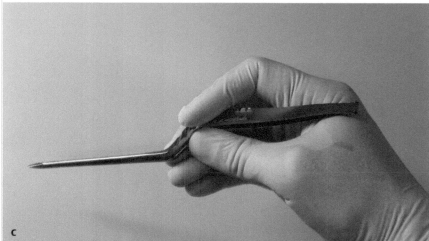

Fig. 3.7 "Index push" technique for holding long bayonet microscissors. The index push technique allows dissection "away from yourself" (vertical cut) (Video 3.10). **(a)** The middle finger is bent in the shape of the bayonet microscissors. It holds the fixed shaft of the instrument at the back edge. The thumb holds this shaft from the other side. **(b)** The forefinger presses down on the moving shaft of the instrument from the top. Only the forefinger moves; the hand and other fingers are fixed. **(c)** This method allows dissection to be performed away from yourself. *Purple arrows* indicate points of contact between the hand and the stable shaft of the instrument; *pink arrows* indicate the motion needed to move the movable shaft of the instrument.

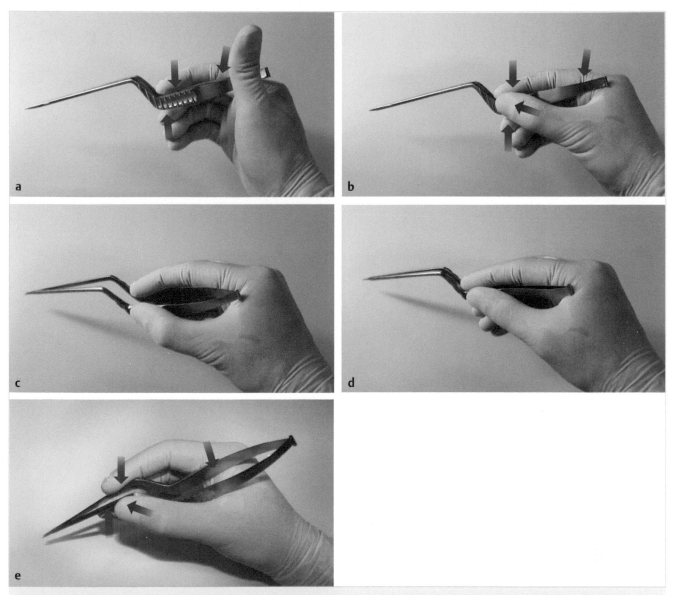

Fig. 3.8 "Chopsticks" technique for holding long bayonet microscissors. The chopsticks technique is used for side-to-side dissection. (Video 3.11). **(a)** In this technique, one shaft is fixed between the index and middle fingers by the edges. **(b)** The thumb is opposed to the index and middle fingers and presses the other shaft of the instrument from the side. Only the thumb moves; the hand and other fingers remain immobile. **(c)** and **(d)** demonstrate the technique for holding scissors in the opened and closed positions, respectively. This technique allows dissection to be performed from either side (i.e., right-to-left or left-to-right dissection). **(e)** For a surface dissection, one usually uses short-handled scissors; however, this handling technique can also be used for a more precise control of the tip of the long instrument. The part of the instrument closer to the tip can be held in the same chopsticks technique. *Purple arrows* indicate points of contact between the hand and the stable shaft of the instrument; *pink arrows* indicate the motion needed to move the movable shaft of the instrument.

3.6 Mastering Dissection with Bayonet Scissors

Effective manipulations with microscissors in a deep operating field demand very precise control of their tips. A glove placed into an empty box (the box the gloves came in is ideal for this exercise) is the first simple model designed to perfect the skills of holding and working with the bayonet scissors.[7] To perform this exercise, you first draw various lines on a glove with a pen and then try to cut the glove within the width of the line (► Fig. 3.10). You must practice changing the position of the instrument, depending on

the direction of the cut, and you must also work with both hands. This exercise will help you to develop a firm and steady scissors-holding technique for dissection in any direction. Mastery of the different individual holding techniques (► Fig. 3.6, ► Fig. 3.7, ► Fig. 3.8) allows the neurosurgeon to perform sharp dissection in almost all possible directions (► Fig. 3.11).

3.7 Warm-up Exercises

After mastering the instrument-holding techniques, you should begin training on the dry models. Do not hesitate to go back

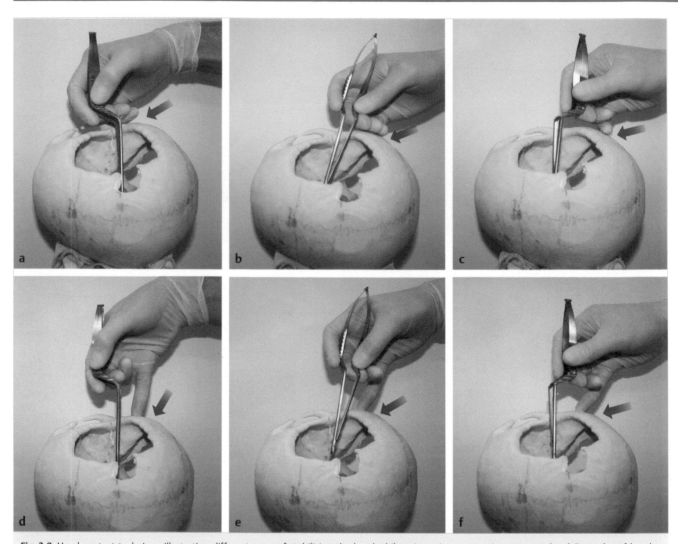

Fig. 3.9 Hand contact technique illustrating different ways of stabilizing the hand while using microsurgery instruments. **(a–c)** Examples of hand contact with the skull when working with short microsurgery instruments or in a deep operational wound. **(d–f)** Examples of contact of the little finger against the skull while working with long instruments or on the surface of an exposure. *Purple arrows* indicate point of contact between fingers and skull.

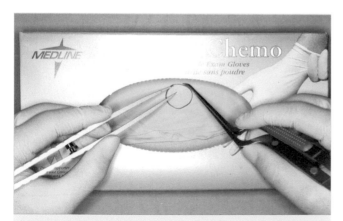

Fig. 3.10 Exercise for practicing different holding techniques and dissection in various directions.

and check different instrument-holding techniques. Holding techniques that initially seemed to be inconvenient may later be advantageous for prolonged work under the microscope, or else they can provide additional maneuverability and steadiness.

The following exercises are initially performed during a 3-hour dry-training practice. Each of these exercises is described more fully below.

1. Knot tying on gauze or on a latex glove: practice all three techniques (i.e., intermittent suture grasping, constant hold of one suture, and constant holding of one suture and pulling in same direction) until you can do each one well (see Sections 3.7.3 through 3.7.5 [p. 37–38]).
2. Untying a knot: practice untying surgical knots (see Section 3.7.8 [p. 40]).
3. End-to-end anastomosis: practice on silicone microtube.
4. End-to-side anastomosis: practice on silicone microtube.
5. Side-to-side anastomosis: practice on silicone microtube.

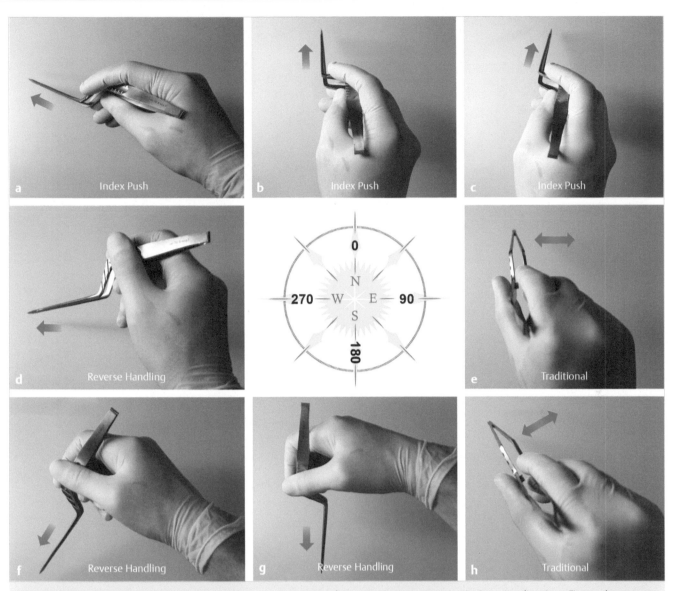

Fig. 3.11 Exercise 1: training in sharp dissection. The compass in center demonstrates "scissors navigation" cutting directions. Figures demonstrate the techniques for holding the bayonet microscissors that are suitable for dissection in these directions (*green arrows*). (**a–c**) The index push technique is used when dissecting in a straight line away from you with the instrument in the upright position or up to 45 degrees to either side. (**d, f, g**) The reverse handling technique is used for dissection toward the left (**d**, 270 degrees), toward the "southwest" (**f**, 225 degrees), and toward the "south" (**g**, 180 degrees). (**e, h**) The traditional technique can be used for straight left-to-right or right-to-left dissection when the instrument is held vertically (**e**) or for dissection angled in a direction from "southwest" to "northeast" when the instrument is held with the tip towards the "northwest" (**h**, 315 degrees).

Perform each of the dry-training exercises first. After that, use a personal set of dry-training exercises to focus on refining specific skills such as tremor control and fast knot tying. For continuous training in your free time, we recommend the following set of exercises (about 10 minutes of total performance time). Each of these exercises is described more fully below.

1. Suturing in different directions (creating a cross or snowflake pattern) (see Section 3.7.7).
2. Untying a knot (see Section 3.7.8).
3. Pushing the end of the suture using the needle tip (see Section 3.7.9).

For the anastomosis training, we recommend routine laboratory practice on tissue models rather than on silicone microtubes. The latter can be used during your initial training while you are memorizing the basic anastomosis principles and sequence of surgical steps. However, silicone has completely different tactile feedback and using it is just a waste of time when tissue models are available instead. When artificial materials are used, microtubes made from new materials have improved elasticity and surface friction compared with silicone, making them more similar to a real cerebral artery and therefore more appropriate for anastomosis training.[8,9]

Short training sessions are enough for acquiring microsurgical skills, but these sessions must be conducted regularly. The optimal approach is to do daily short morning sessions consisting of 10 sutures on gauze by the left and right hands (cross or snowflake).[6] The training exercises should also be varied from time to time because conditions in the operating room vary: simulate manipulations in a deep surgical wound, practice suturing on gauze in different directions, practice anastomoses on elastic tubes, and practice anastomoses on live tissues.

3.7.1 Knot Tying on Gauze

Tying knots on gauze is one of the first fundamental exercises (▶ Fig. 3.12). Continuous repetition of this exercise is essential for obtaining needle- and suture-handling skills. Even the experienced neurosurgeon may need to refresh and maintain this skill.[10]

To master suturing, you must be able to suture in all directions with both hands. In clinical situations, the tissues must be oriented, as much as possible, so that the manipulations can be maximally productive and convenient.

In most cases, a sailor's knot is tied, which is more secure than a "granny knot." A surgical knot, which is made by forming two unilateral loops, is used as a first knot when it is necessary to keep the sutured tissues under tension without the suture coming undone while preparing the second throw. A sailor's knot made up of three throws of the suture is usually enough for making a single complete tie when suturing microscale vessels.

In the beginning stage, it is easier to grasp a needle with forceps using the technique depicted in ▶ Fig. 3.13.

Knots can be tied using any of the various techniques. The technique that enables you to maintain constant hold of one suture end is the quickest and is applied in clinical practice more often than other techniques. Naturally, the quickest and most effective surgery is achieved by avoiding unnecessary and nonproductive movements.

3.7.2 Notes about Suturing

Suturing is performed under high magnification (20× to 30×) to enable you to best visualize the vessel wall, whereas tying knots may be performed under low magnification (10×) to enable you to best visualize the ends of ligatures and form loops. With more experience, you can perform everything under high magnification, which saves time.

One suture needle may be used several times during a training exercise, with the suture shortening after each knot. However, the more it is used, the more the needle becomes dull and the suture material becomes damaged. The suture is very thin and fragile, and it is easily deformed, bent, frayed, and, eventually, torn. For this reason, 9–0 and 10–0 sutures are not reused multiple times during surgery.

Microsurgical suturing is the basis of microsurgical training; hence, you should repeat these exercises as often as possible to practice your suturing skill, and once mastered, they should be repeated as often as possible to refresh your skill. Despite being acquired in the laboratory, this microsurgical skill does not differ much from that required under real operating room conditions, despite additional challenges such as the presence of blood and the need to maintain aseptic conditions.

In the laboratory setting, you should always train in surgical gloves, so as to better simulate conditions in the operating room. There are distinct tactile differences between suturing with naked hands and suturing with gloved hands. Under some surgical conditions, double-gloving may be necessary. However, when performing microanastomoses, a single layer of glove allows better tactile feedback, and special gloves for microsurgery are also available.

Knot tying is a crucial step at the end of the suturing process. Knots should be tight; light should not be visible through a knot. Knots should be fully secure. The three different knot-tying methods are described below. A very important point is that the described knot-tying methods will not work unless you grab the suture thread appropriately at the very begining. When you grab the suture, you should make sure that the looping segment of the suture forms an obtuse angle with the forceps (as shown in ▶ Fig. 3.14b and ▶ Fig. 3.15b). During knot formation, the instruments should not cross or touch each other; rather, one instrument directs the movements of the loop around the opposite instrument.

3.7.3 Knot-Tying Method 1: Intermittent Suture Grasping

The first knot-tying method produces a secure sailor's knot and is based on intermittent grasping of the sutures with the forceps (▶ Fig. 3.14). Because releasing and recapturing the suture requires more time, this method takes longer than other methods. For this reason, it is not the most frequently used method in actual operations. However, early in your training, it is a useful method to practice. This method familiarizes you with the small-scale haptics of a tiny needle and suture, as you begin to experience how it feels to form the loops and to grasp the small sutures with forceps.

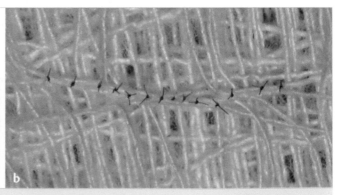

Fig. 3.12 Exercise 2: tying knots on gauze. (a) Insertion of needle through the neighboring gauze fibers. (b) A series of completed knots.

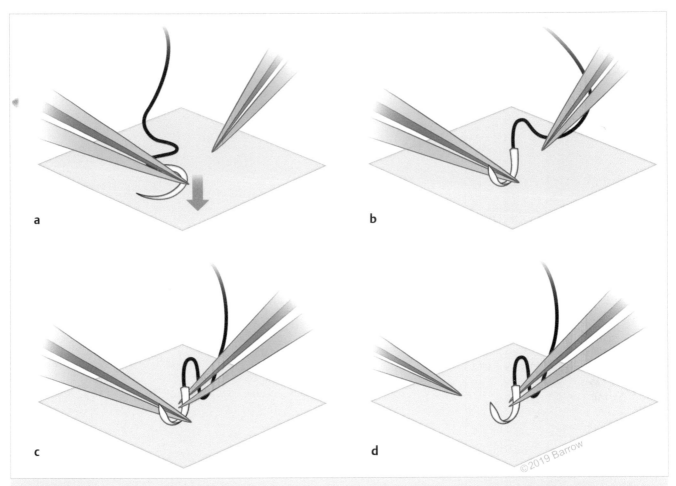

Fig. 3.13 Technique for picking up a needle from a flat surface. **(a)** Push down on the center of the needle with the left forceps. **(b)** The needle turns by itself, so the point and shaft are directed upward. **(c)** Grasp the needle with the forceps and **(d)** remove the left forceps (Video 3.12).

3.7.4 Knot-Tying Method 2: Constant Hold of One Suture

The second knot-tying method decreases the time required to produce a knot because one suture is permanently held by the forceps and unnecessary manipulations are avoided (▶ Fig. 3.15). Due to the elasticity of the monofilament, this suture has a shape memory. Thus, a simple linear motion of the instrument with the suture makes it form a loop and makes tying the knot easier. At least three antiparallel throws are needed to make a reliable knot with a thin (9–0 or 10–0) monofilament, but usually four antiparallel throws are performed for safety. Two tricks can help minimize the force and the time required to complete a knot: (1) choose an appropriate length of the suture end to grasp by the forceps before making a knot; and (2) always place and operate the forceps near the formed loop and puncture site to avoid far-reaching movements. Every time you release a suture from the forceps, you lose time and increase emotional tension, and these factors can influence the surgical outcome. Be careful not to break the long end of the suture during tightening, because when the suture bends around the instrument, it becomes fragile and may later rupture at the weakened point.

3.7.5 Knot-Tying Method 3: Constant Hold of One Suture and Pulling in the Same Direction

The third knot-tying method is a modification of the second method. A sliding knot is formed, depending on the direction of tightening when using this method (▶ Fig. 3.16). This knot is not as reliable as a sailor's knot. However, this method can be successfully applied in surgical procedures, and it has a distinct advantage in that the short end of the suture is always tightened in the same direction—toward yourself—that may be useful in a deep operative field.

3.7.6 Method of Simultaneous Cutting of Suture Tails

Cut the ends of the sutures with microscissors. They can be cut one after another by stretching them with the forceps. But you can accelerate the process and save time by holding up the two sutures together with one forceps to allow simultaneous cutting of the ends (▶ Fig. 3.17).

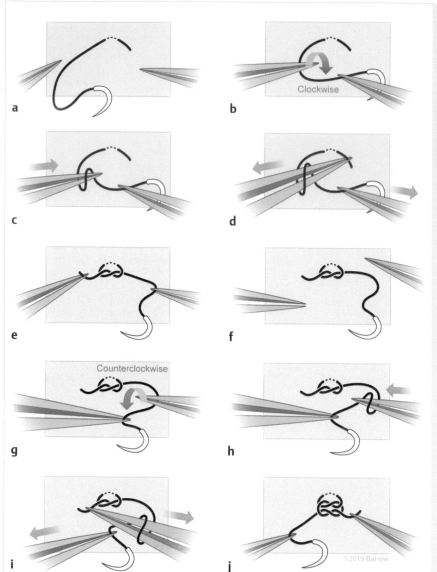

Fig. 3.14 Knot-tying method 1: intermittent suture grasping. Three consecutive knots are formed by following these steps. (*Arrows* show motion of forceps.) **(a)** The forceps are placed opposite one another (the left forceps near the long end of the suture, the right forceps near the short end). **(b)** The long end of the suture (on the left) is grasped by the right forceps, and a loop is formed around the left forceps with a clockwise looping motion of the right forceps. **(c)** The short end of the suture is grasped by the left forceps. **(d)** The knot is tightened (the right forceps pulls to the right, and the left forceps pulls to the left). **(e)** After the knot is completed, the ends of the suture can be released. **(f)** To form the second knot, first, the long end of the suture (now on the right) is grasped by the left forceps. **(g)** A loop is then formed around the right forceps with a counterclockwise looping motion of the left forceps. **(h)** The short end of the suture is grasped by the right forceps and **(i)** pulled to the right, and **(j)** the knot is tightened (the right forceps pulls to the right, and the left forceps pulls to the left). The ends of the suture are then released. The third knot (*not shown*) is formed in the same way as the first knot (Video 3.13).

3.7.7 The "Snowflake" Exercise

The needle-passing motion should be mastered in all directions. Ideally, both hands should be trained to make needle passes. The following exercise is designed to train you in holding and passing the needle gently and purposefully in all possible directions (▶ Fig. 3.18). Two or three separate sutures should be oriented in all 8 directions, for a total of 16 to 24 stiches. Vessels will not always lie down in an alignment comfortable for suturing, so developing the ability to hold and pass the needle is invaluable.

> ### Sidebar
>
> In the beginning, your manipulations of the microsurgery instruments under the microscope will be rather slow. However, you will become faster with practice. Learning how to generate smooth and accurate movements is the priority. Once you can consistently produce smooth and accurate movements, you can then focus on improving your speed.

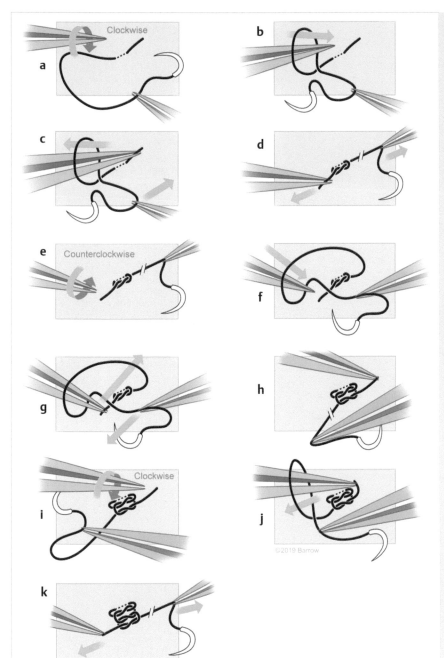

Fig. 3.15 Knot-tying method 2: constant hold of one suture. (*Arrows* show motion of forceps.) **(a)** The right forceps grasps the long end of the suture and is moved to the place of puncture. A loop is formed by a looping move of the right forceps around the left forceps, and **(b)** the left forceps is moved through the loop to grasp the distal short end of the suture. **(c)** The forceps with the distal end of the suture (on the left) is moved toward you, and the forceps with the long end with the needle (on the right, proximal end) is moved away from you. **(d)** Tighten the knot by gently pulling the ends as shown. When the knot is tightened, the suture stretches and the ends stay in the same position. (*Short parallel lines* on suture show that length of suture is longer than can be shown in image.) **(e)** The right forceps with the long end of the suture is not released, and the looping motion is repeated around the left forceps at the place of puncture to form a loop. **(f)** The left forceps is moved through the loop. **(g)** The short end of the suture is grasped by the left forceps and is pulled up, while the long end is pulled down with the right forceps **(h)** forming the second knot. The knot is tightened by gently pulling the suture ends aside as shown. **(i–k)** The third knot is formed in the same manner as the first knot. The right forceps should constantly hold the long end of the suture while performing all throws and tightening (Video 3.14).

3.7.8 Untying a Knot

In this exercise, first tie 10 sequential sailor's knots using the 10–0 suture on the fibers of a piece of gauze. Your task is to untie the knots one by one using microforceps and a needle (▶ Fig. 3.19). You may exercise untying with both the right and left hands to train for dexterity.

3.7.9 Pushing the Suture End

This exercise teaches you how to relax and remain calm because the exercise can only be done with the absolute absence of tremor. The task is to push the end of the suture thread with the tip of the suture needle so that it passes through the gauze fiber (▶ Fig. 3.20). A new 10–0 suture must

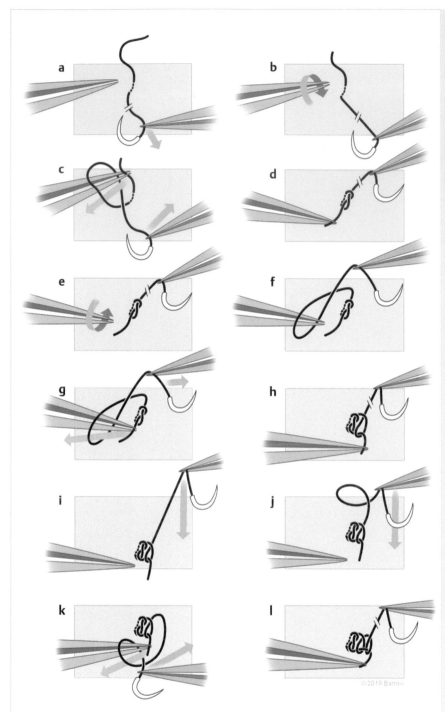

Fig. 3.16 Knot-tying method 3: constant hold of one suture and tightening in a single direction. **(a)** Starting position. The left forceps tips are positioned near the puncture site ready to grasp the short tail end. The tail end is intentionally left longer initially (the estimated length should include the final length of the suture tail plus the final length of the long looping end). Then the long end is grasped with the right forceps near the puncture site and pulled until the tail end becomes the appropriate (short) length. (*Short parallel lines* on suture show that length of suture is longer than can be shown in image.) This maneuver allows you to grasp the long end at the place where it can be seen more clearly. From this moment on, the right forceps constantly holds the long end of the suture without releasing it. **(b)** A looping motion is used to move the right forceps around the left forceps to form a loop. **(c)** The left forceps is moved through the loop to grasp the short end of the suture, and the ends are pulled in the directions shown (*arrows*). **(d)** The knot is tightened. The resulting first knot and forceps position is shown. **(e)** The short end of the suture is then released from the left forceps and the right forceps is moved down with a looping motion around the left forceps. **(f)** The resulting loop is shown. **(g)** The short end of the suture is grasped with the left forceps and pulled through the loop, as shown on the figure. **(h)** The resulting sliding knot and the position of the instruments are shown. It is important not to release or weaken the grasp of the right forceps on the long suture end at this moment. **(i)** The suture is released from the left forceps. The right forceps is moved down toward the place of puncture. **(j)** Note that the long suture end automatically forms a loop. **(k)** The left forceps are continued to be moved down while the suture forms a loop until the loop is near the short end. The left forceps is then inserted through the loop to grasp the short end. The ends are pulled in opposite directions as shown (*arrows*). **(l)** The resulting knot is tightened by pulling the suture ends. After the knot is completed, the ends of the sutures are trimmed (*not shown*) (Video 3.15).

©2019 Barrow

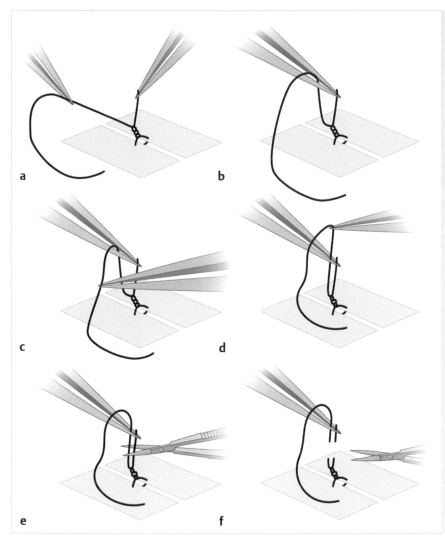

Fig. 3.17 Simultaneous cutting of the suture tails. **(a)** The final knot is tightened by pulling the suture ends to each side. **(b)** The left forceps grasps the short end (tail) of the suture, so that the longer suture end stays in between the shafts of the forceps. **(c)** The right forceps grasps the longer tail of the suture and lifts it up. **(d)** The longer suture end is pulled up to move it closer to the short end. Closing the left forceps tighter enables you to hold the two tails of the suture with a single forceps. **(e, f)** Exchange the instrument in the right hand for microscissors and cut the two tails of the suture at the same time.

be used for this exercise because the scissors flatten the end of the suture as they cut, which makes the end of the suture too sharp to push with the needle tip.

Sidebar

To master microsurgical technique, you will need to get used to the types of microsurgery instruments and to the "micro-world" with its own laws of physics. Learn how to relax the muscles of your back, shoulders, arms, and hands. Feeling relaxed is difficult, especially at the beginning, but with training you can learn how to do it over time. Professional musicians and athletes say that the most important factor for good performance is the absence of tension in their muscles, and this point is equally true for microneurosurgery.

The "untying a knot" and "pushing the suture end" exercises are difficult but not impossible to perform if you can get your muscles relaxed enough. These exercises can also help you to learn how to maintain mental control and relax your muscles.

3.8 Anastomosis on a "Dry" Model

In neurosurgery, anastomoses are divided into direct and indirect. Direct anastomoses are formed by joining vessel lumens; the three types are *end-to-end*, *end-to-side*, and *side-to-side* anastomoses (▶ Fig. 3.21). Indirect anastomoses are formed independently by the de novo formation of the vessels. Basic techniques of direct anastomoses are described in this chapter, whereas nuances are discussed later in Chapter 5, in the section on live tissue models.

3.8.1 Anastomosis on Synthetic Microtubes

Silicone tubes can be used as a type of artificial vessel in the beginning stages of microsurgical training (▶ Fig. 3.22). They can help you to understand the main principles of performing anastomoses. Working with the tubes can elicit interest in microvascular neurosurgery. However, the elastic properties of the tubes do not correspond to those of live tissues, which is why they cannot replace wet training.

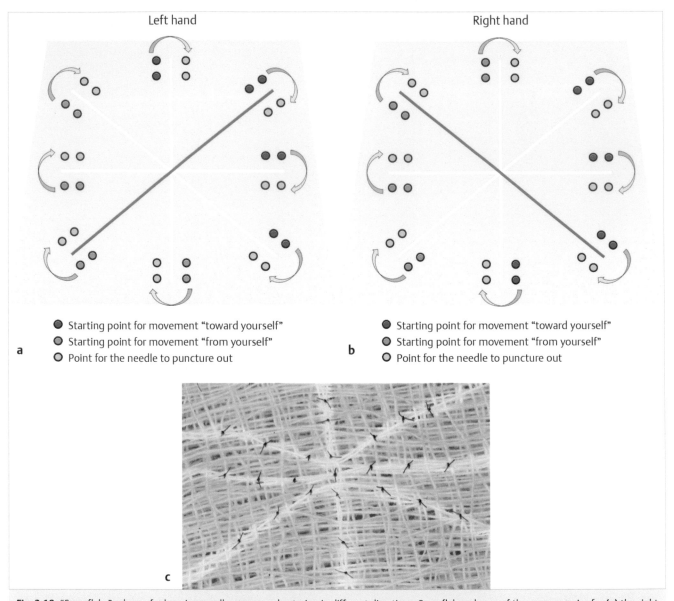

Fig. 3.18 "Snowflake" schema for learning needle passes and suturing in different directions. Snowflake schema of the same exercise for **(a)** the right hand and **(b)** the left hand. *Blue line* represents the most comfortable position for suturing edges. *Colored dots* represent the places for the needle to go "in" (*red and orange dots*) and "out" (*blue dots*). The suturing can be done on a piece of surgical gauze or a latex glove. **(c)** Final result after completing snowflake suturing exercise on surgical gauze with 10–0 suture.

Silicone tubes are manufactured in different sizes and are available from industrial supply stores. In addition, training cards (microvascular practice card, Muranaka medical instruments Co., Ltd., Osaka, Japan) (▶ Fig. 3.22a) are available for practice suturing.[11] For microsurgery practice, 8–0, 9–0, and 10–0 sutures are usually used for tubes with diameters of 2.0, 1.0, and 0.7 mm, respectively. For supermicrosurgery (surgery on vessels 0.5 mm or smaller), 11–0 and 12–0 sutures are used for tubes with diameters of 0.5 or 0.3 mm. The cost of a set in 2016 was about US $50 to $80. Another material, polyvinyl alcohol (PVA) hydrogel, appeared to have better qualities than silicone for simulation of the properties of the human cerebral arteries. These tubes (KEZLEX, Ono and Co., Ltd., Tokyo, Japan) (▶ Fig. 3.22c) are also readily available for purchase at a cost of about US $120.[9] Different simulators based on synthetic microtubes are also widely used in microsurgical training, such as a microvascular simulator[12] or MD-PVC Rat Model (Braintree Scientific, Inc., Braintree, Massachusetts, USA). Despite the criticism, silicone tubes, especially PVA hydrogel tubes, are helpful for learning the counter-press method (▶ Fig. 3.23) (described in Section 3.8.3), as well as for learning suturing techniques and knot-tying techniques in different directions.

3.8.2 Anastomosis on a Latex Glove

If microtubes are not available, a latex glove can be used. A thin leaf made from a latex or nitrile glove, which simulates a wall of

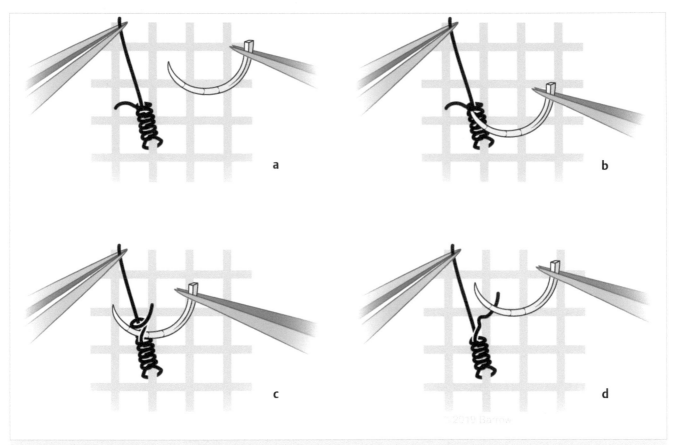

Fig. 3.19 Exercise 4: untying a knot. **(a)** Use the left forceps to hold the longer end of the suture in tension. **(b)** Grasp the needle in the right forceps and try to insert the needle inside the knot. **(c)** After the needle point has been successfully inserted in the knot, pull it up to untie the knot. **(d)** The upper knot has been untied (Video 3.16).

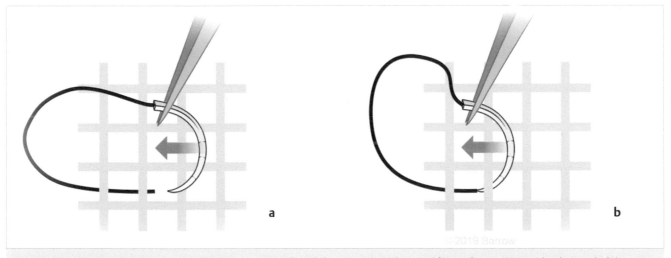

Fig. 3.20 Exercise 5: pushing the suture end. **(a)** First, sequentially pull the suture through several fibers of gauze, leaving the short end of the suture near the first fiber. **(b)** With the tip of the needle, push the tail end of the suture smoothly forward through the gauze fiber (Video 3.17).

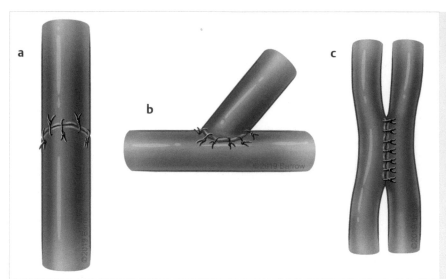

Fig. 3.21 Types of direct anastomoses. (a) End-to-end anastomosis. (b) End-to-side anastomosis. (c) Side-to-side anastomosis.

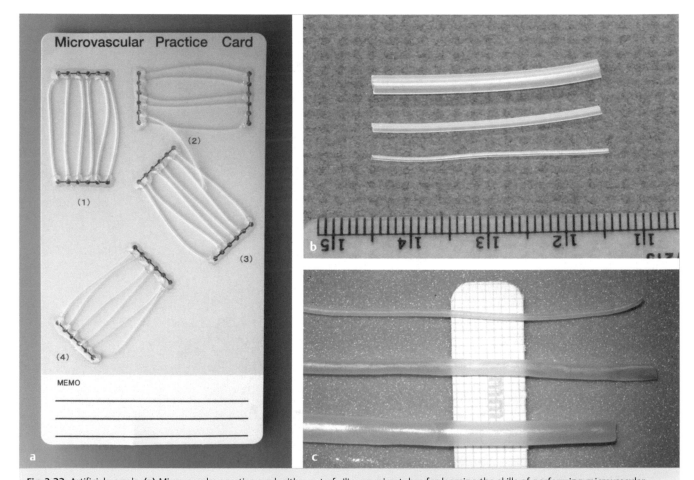

Fig. 3.22 Artificial vessels. (a) Microvascular practice card with a set of silicone microtubes for learning the skills of performing microvascular anastomoses. (b) Silicone tubes of various diameters can be purchased separately in any desirable length. (c) Polyvinyl alcohol (PVA) hydrogel tubes with surface friction, transparency, and elasticity properties that are qualitatively similar to those of human vessels. However, PVA tubes are more expensive than silicone and dry out quickly.

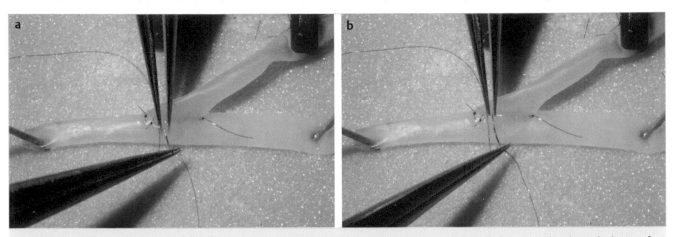

Fig. 3.23 Simulation of end-to-side anastomosis on silicone microtubes. **(a)** Counter-press method. The upper forceps is placed into the lumen of a vessel and exerts pressure from inside, while the lower forceps is pushing the needle from outside. **(b)** The upper forceps are slightly opened and exert pressure from outside, while the needle is pushed from inside.

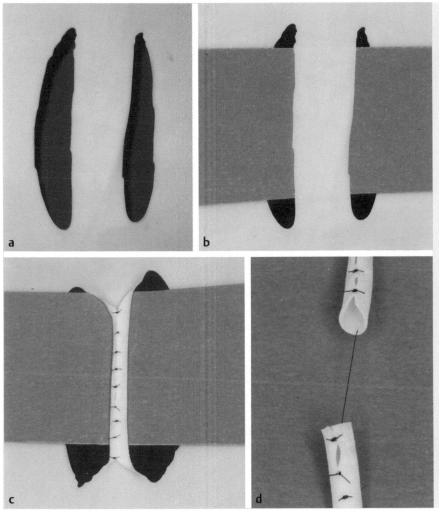

Fig. 3.24 Exercise 3: training on a latex glove. The glove is stretched out and fixed on a flat surface using adhesive tape. **(a)** First, make two parallel cuts on the glove. **(b)** A strip of blue background paper is inserted through the vertical cuts. **(c)** Then, suture the inner edges together to form a tube ("vessel"). **(d)** Next, cut the tube in half, to perform end-to-end anastomosis.

microvessels, can help you to practice suturing. The thickness of the leaf is about 120–170 μm (▶ Fig. 3.24). Examination gloves are also elastic, so when tightening the knot, you will find that the suture does not seem to be clearly in focus at all times. All three knot-tying methods should be mastered initially. Doing so will help you to learn the properties of the thread of the 9–0 and 10–0 sutures and their tactile feedback. Ultimately, you will select the fastest knot-tying method for surgery and use the other methods less frequently to handle difficult positions. Practicing microsuturing on an examination glove or a surgical glove is also useful for helping you to adapt to the changes in the optimal focal distance as you tighten sutures in different directions and under different angles of view.

3.8.3 Types of Suturing Techniques

Interrupted Suturing Technique

When you are performing a vascular suture, the needle puncture should remain perpendicular to the vessel wall surface, some distance in from the edge. Use the counter-press technique to push the needle between the branches of the forceps so that you can grasp it with them after loosening the needle from the needle holder. Then pull the needle out far enough to be able to grasp it at the body part with the needle holder. Next, grasp the opposite vessel wall with the forceps and lift it. The needle punctures the opposite side, just in from the edge, from inside the vessel lumen, and importantly, is directed upward

(i.e., perpendicular to the vessel wall). Release the grasp of the needle holder on the needle and take out the suture with the forceps. When you pull out the suture, leave a short end that is still long enough to make a knot. Then tie the knot.

Counter-Press Method

The counter-press method is used to facilitate the puncture of the vessel wall with the needle (▶ Fig. 3.25). Bring the microforceps inside the vessel lumen. Then, with the branches of the forceps slightly opened, apply counterpressure to the inside of the vessel wall so that the needle will puncture the wall and go between the blades of the forceps. You should avoid intima exfoliation and uneven capturing of the vessel wall.

Suturing from the inside out is performed by raising the vessel wall with the forceps by gently grasping the periadventitial sheath of the vessel (▶ Fig. 3.26). This way of suturing promotes

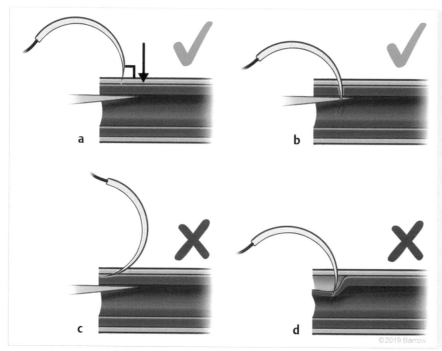

Fig. 3.25 The counter-press method: suturing from the outside. (a) The puncturing of all the layers of the vessel wall should be done at a right angle. (b) Counterpressure on the wall of the vessel from the inside by the forceps. (c) Wrong: uneven capturing of the vessel wall. (d) Wrong: exfoliation of the intima can occur if the forceps are not used for counterpressure.

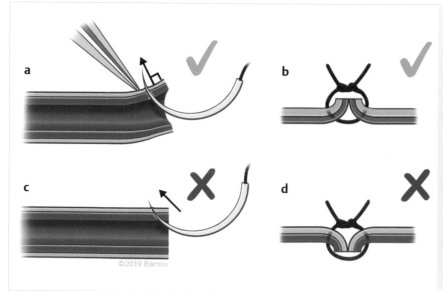

Fig. 3.26 The counter-press method: suturing from the inside. (a) The puncture of the needle in the vessel wall must be completely perpendicular, which is facilitated by raising the wall of the vessel with the forceps. (b) Coaptation of the "intima-intima" layer after the knot is tied. (c) Wrong: uneven capturing of the vessel wall. (d) Wrong: folding the vessel wall inside the lumen.

better matching of the intimal layers of the vessels. You should avoid uneven capturing of the vessel wall, and you should avoid folding the vessel edges back inside, which may cause thrombosis.

Running to Interrupted Suturing Technique

Suturing can also be performed using the original method: make running sutures and leave a loose loop of suture after each stitch. Then cut the loops with microscissors and tie the resulting ends of the sutures in pairs to make a series of interrupted sutures (▶ Fig. 3.27). This method may save time during the process of suturing.[17,18]

Another variation is to cut the loop after each needle pass. When small-size sutures are used (10–0, 9–0, or 8–0), you can save time by actually tearing the suture loop with two forceps instead of exchanging one instrument for scissors. Then tie the resultant suture ends one by one to create a series of interrupted sutures.

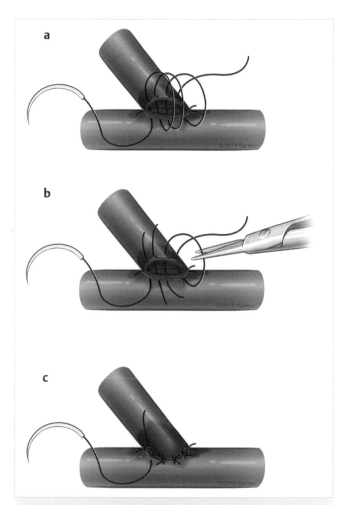

Fig. 3.27 Running-to-interrupted vascular suture technique for end-to-side anastomosis. (a) First, make loose running sutures to keep the lumen opened and prevent it from becoming deformed. This technique facilitates the placement of each needle pass and the selection of evenly spaced intervals between the sutures (b). After the loose running sutures are placed, cut the thread loops. (c) Finalize the anastomosis by tying the cut loops to form interrupted sutures.

Running Suturing Technique

The technique known as *running suturing* is more popular in the US, while interrupted suturing is more common in Japan. The most common reason for not using the running technique is limited widening of the vessels and even potential narrowing of the lumen. It is rarely used for small microvascular anastomoses, but it can be applied when the attaching vessel lumens are more than 1.5 mm in diameter. Running sutures can be safely used for the following:

1. Closing the arteriotomy
2. Large end-to-end anastomoses when the free end of the vessel is short (e.g., when it is impossible to rotate the vessel, you can suture the back lip of the anastomosis using a running suture beginning with the inner side and then placing interrupted sutures on the outer side).
3. Side-to-side anastomosis
4. End-to-side anastomosis

A disadvantage of the running suture is the possibility of corrugating the wall of the vessel when tying a knot. Another disadvantage is the possibility of pulling the suture insufficiently tight, so the whole line of sutures is loose. The risk of narrowing the vessel lumen is especially undesirable when performing an end-to-end anastomosis; therefore, interrupted suturing is usually preferable for this type of anastomosis.

3.8.4 Types of Anastomosis

End-to-End Anastomosis

An end-to-end anastomosis is typically used in microsurgical restorative operations. The orifices of the anastomosed vessels must have identical diameters. The "clock" principle will help you to accurately approximate the vessels. For convenience, imagine dividing the circumference of the vessel wall into 12 identical parts, as on a clock face. Such division will help you to estimate the number of interrupted sutures needed and the distance between them. The first stiches are performed on the upper side, at 10 and 2 o'clock (using the eccentric biangulation method of Cobbett[13]) (▶ Fig. 3.28). If the sutures were to be performed opposite one another (at 3 and 9 o'clock), the top and bottom walls of the vessel would collapse.[14] If that happens, it will be difficult to create a space between the collapsed walls and to puncture the right place in the vessel wall without damaging or catching the opposite wall. If the connecting vessel ends are under tension, the first knot can be a surgical one (two loops), or a granny's knot (slip knot), which enables retention of the vessel attached during the formation of the next securing sailor's knots.

After applying two stay sutures, rotate the temporary clips 180 degrees, so that the vessel is twisted, showing the bottom side. The appropriate position of traction sutures ensures a slightly released anastomosis opening. Place the third suture at the 6 o'clock position. Then place the rest of the sutures equidistant around the face of the clock.

A stepwise end-to-end anastomosis exercise is shown in ▶ Fig. 3.29. Unlike silicone tubes, which are relatively rigid and stay open during the creation of an anastomosis, real vessels will collapse. To prevent the collapse, you may perform stay sutures by using the eccentric biangulation method,[13] with the stay sutures held in place by slits in the colored latex lining

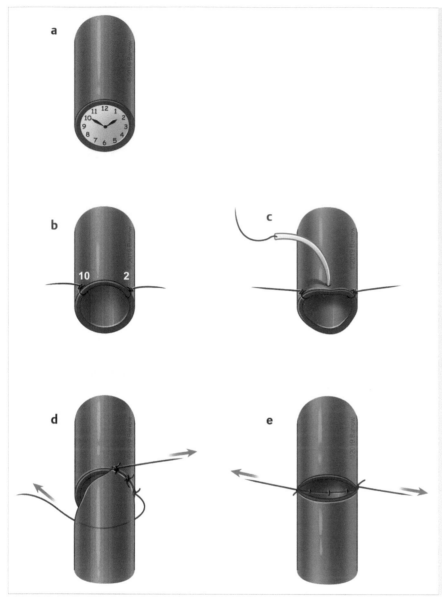

Fig. 3.28 Creating an end-to-end anastomosis. **(a)** The "clock" principle for determining the position on the vessel's circumference. **(b)** Perform stay sutures by using the eccentric biangulation method of Cobbett,[13] leave the ends of the sutures long enough to pull them aside and secure in this position (second vessel not shown). **(c)** Suture the front semicircumference of the anastomosis. **(d, e)** Rotate the vessels by traction on the first two sutures, and then suture the back semicircumference of anastomosis.

background (▶ Fig. 3.30). This helps to maintain tension on the orifice of the anastomosis.

End-to-Side Anastomosis

The end-to-side anastomosis is used most often in neurosurgical practice. It is used for direct extraintracranial bypass procedures and intracranial in situ vascular reconstructions. Thus, most of your training time should be devoted to this type of anastomosis. The steps in performing an end-to-side anastomosis are as follows:

1. Preparation of the donor and recipient vessels
2. Piercing the "heel" and the "toe" of the donor vessel with traction sutures
3. Applying temporary clips on recipient vessel and performing the arteriotomy
4. Forming the anastomosis
5. Checking the quality of the anastomosis

Different configurations of the donor vessel can be used to create the end-to-side anastomosis (▶ Fig. 3.31). The various possible geometries of the anastomosed vessel are important for their effect on the vessel's rheological properties, and thus the chosen geometry is one of the factors contributing to the long-term patency of the anastomosis. Other important parameters of anastomosis are the angle between the donor vessel and the recipient vessel, the size of the vessels, and the bends and kinks of the donor vessel before anastomosing.[15] The angle and the shape of the cutting pattern vary. Depending on the aim of the anastomosis, the structure of the vessel, the thickness of the vessel wall, the vessel diameter, and the gradient of blood flow, you can use different cutting patterns of the donor vessel and recipient vessel, such as diamond-shaped or rounded. Silicone microtubes stay open continuously and thus are perfect substrates to try different tailoring methods for the donor vessel.

The fish-mouth technique to tailor the donor vessel is commonly used in microsurgery because it results in a widely

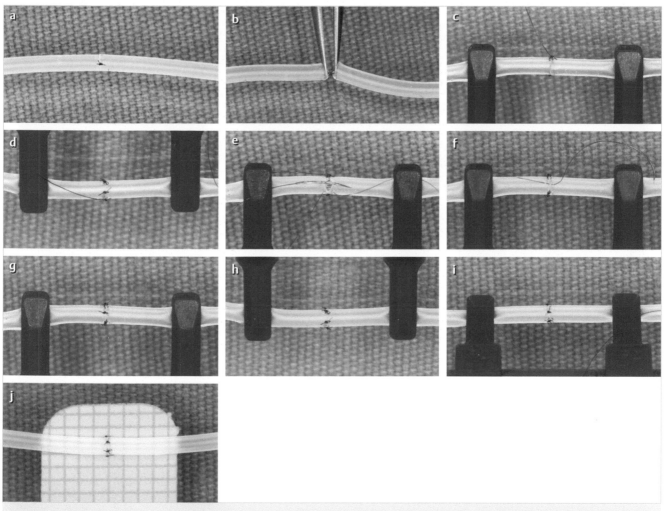

Fig. 3.29 Stepwise creation of an end-to-end anastomosis on a 1-mm diameter silicone microtube. **(a)** The ends of the tube are aligned in an end-to-end fashion and secured with a single 10–0 suture. **(b)** In this view, the first suture is shown from inside, while the silicone vessels are pulled away with gentle opening of the forceps. Note the stiff nature of the silicone. Take care not to push the needle, suture, or vessel too hard to prevent unintended wall cuts. **(c)** The ends of the vessel are fixed in place with two opposing sutures. Leaving one long suture tail will facilitate the choice of needle puncture points later on. You can pull this suture end to distend the vessel wall. **(d)** Microvascular clips with approximator (apppproximator connecting two clips is not shown) are then rotated 180 degrees, and two interrupted sutures are made in the back wall. **(e)** The approximator is rotated back exposing the front wall. The back wall is checked from the inside for loose sutures. **(f)** Two interrupted sutures are placed on the front wall. **(g)** Completed anastomosis. **(h)** Approximator is rotated away to check the back wall again. **(i)** View from the side (initial side stay suture). Pay attention, as it is a common place to make sutures unevenly with unequal distance from the neighboring sutures, which can result in bleeding or narrowing of the artery. **(j)** View of the completed anastomosis on a millimeter-gridded paper dam.

opened anastomotic lumen (▶ Fig. 3.32). In creating the fish-mouth opening, you should accurately align the walls of the vessels without creating excess tension. A considerable part of the wall of the anastomosis is provided by the donor vessel; it lies prone and "hugs" the recipient vessel, allowing an increase in blood flow through the anastomosis and thereby decreasing the possibility of thrombosis. Another practical note during fish-mouth anastomosis: if the anastomosis is tailored so that the oblique cut is the same length as the longitudinal cut (as shown in ▶ Fig. 3.32a), then the sharp turn of the donor vessel anastomosis line will be located exactly at the midpoint of its total length. Knowing this principle helps to fashion an arteriotomy of the appropriate length and to find the precise position to put a middle suture between the toe and heel sutures.

You can perform the incision on a recipient vessel in several ways. First, you can make a linear incision by using a no. 11 surgical blade or the 30-gauge needle tip of an insulin syringe. Second, you can apply a single stay suture to the vessel wall, which you then use to lift the wall, while performing an oval arteriotomy with curved microscissors. The arteriotomy can also be performed with microscissors or with special microscissors with an angulated vertical cut mechanism.

To avoid corrugation and to support the wall, a short fragment of a silastic tube can be inserted into the recipient vessel before suturing and removed before the final suture is secured.[16] Suturing is usually performed the standard way. You make the first suture from the "heel" of the anastomosis and the second from the "toe." Then you make the interrupted

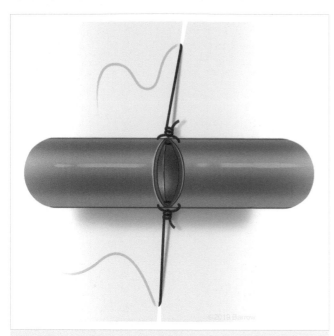

Fig. 3.30 Traction sutures can be held in place in slits in the colored latex lining.

sutures on one side of the anastomosis. Turn the donor vessel when necessary to check from the inside whether the opposite wall was unintentionally caught in a suture. In order to leave space for counter-press from inside the lumen, the last two sutures are made in the following way: prick the walls of the vessels as in a running suture, check the inner surface of the anastomosed vessel, then cut the loops and form single interrupted sutures one after another.

In performing an arterial anastomosis, you should make the puncture of the needle at a distance from the edge that is equal to or twice as much as the thickness of the artery. In venous anastomosis, you should make the puncture at a distance of about twice the thickness of the vein.

Use the counter-press method to make the needle puncture. First, place semi-opened forceps into the vessel lumen to press the wall from the inside toward the needle puncture. Applying counterpressure this way will help to save the opposite wall of the vessel from excessive tension and from tearing at the place of puncture, and it also prevents formation of intimal flap. Moreover, it allows you to grasp the needle by the forceps to pull the suture out. Puncturing the vessel wall from inside out also prevents intimal flap detachment.

Side-to-Side Anastomosis

In rare clinical situations, you will need to form a side-to-side anastomosis. To create a side-to-side anastomosis, place two temporary clips to bring the vessels close together and occlude flow. Stabilize each vessel to avoid excess tension with a pair of microclips. After approximation of the walls of the vessel, perform the arteriotomies on both vessels. The back wall is

sutured through all the layers with a running suture first. The key initial maneuver after completion of the first stay suture is to pass the needle from the outer side of the vessel in between them at the site of the arteriotomy and to pass the needle from outside to inside on the correct vessel. This step is important because it sets up the direction of suturing: toward yourself or away from yourself. You should puncture the lower vessel (in horizontally oriented vessels) or the left vessel (in vertically oriented vessels) to proceed with suturing toward yourself with your right hand. Then use a running suture to secure the opposite edges of the arteriotomies.

There are two methods for placing stay sutures. One method is to first perform two stay sutures at the ends of the anastomosis and then to perform the running suture between them from inside the vessel. This method is good, but it brings two vessels so close to each other that passing the needle between them can be difficult. An alternate method is to place only one stay suture to secure the position of the vessels. Not using a second stay suture provides more space for movement of the instrument between the vessels, which makes suturing easier using a counter-press method. Using one stay suture makes possible three possible variants for finishing the first side of the anastomosis.

1. Finish the running row using the same suture, and perform the knot between the last loop and the suture tail.
2. Make a second stay suture with a separate suture thread, and tie the tail of the first suture to it. Suturing the opposite side can be continued starting from the second stay suture.
3. Continue suturing the front wall of the anastomosis with the same suture without making a stay suture (not recommended due to the risk of narrowing).

The advantage of placing a second stay suture is that it provides additional tightening of the running suture after the final suturing is finished. Without such a stay suture, the risk is higher for vessel corrugation due to overtraction of the suturing thread. The front wall can be sutured with either running or interrupted sutures.

A stepwise description of the side-to-side anastomosis technique on silicone microtubes is presented in ▶ Fig. 3.33.

Repairing a Ruptured Suture

If the needle tears out of the suture or the suture tears in the middle of the running suture, the suturing can still be repaired (▶ Fig. 3.34). You should make sure that the torn tail is facing outside the vessel and is of sufficient length to be grabbed to form a knot. Then continue suturing from the same point but at the opposite side of the anastomosis with a new suture. Pass the new needle (suture) from the outside of the vessel to the inside, leaving a tail to tie to the torn tail. When you reach the toe or heel of the anastomosis with the new suture, secure it in a knot using the last loop and the suture tail. Then tighten the torn tail from the first suture with the tail of the new suture from outside the vessel lumen and secure them with a knot. This method allows you to repair a running suture and suspend tension equally between the two threads. It also prevents over-tension or loosening of the running suture.

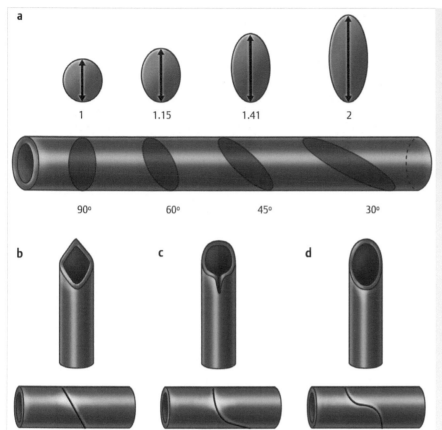

Fig. 3.31 Shapes of donor vessel orifices. **(a)** The coefficient (1, 1.15, 1.41, 2) by which the longer diameter of the vessel orifice is enlarging, depending on the angle of the cut. For example, a 30-degree cut produces an orifice that is twice as large as that produced by a 90-degree straight perpendicular vessel cut. **(b)** A straight cut produces a sharp angular tip at the toe-side of the donor vessel. **(c)** A hockey-stick shaped cut produces a sharp angle at the heel of the donor vessel. **(d)** An oblique loose S-shaped cut produces an oval orifice in the donor vessel.

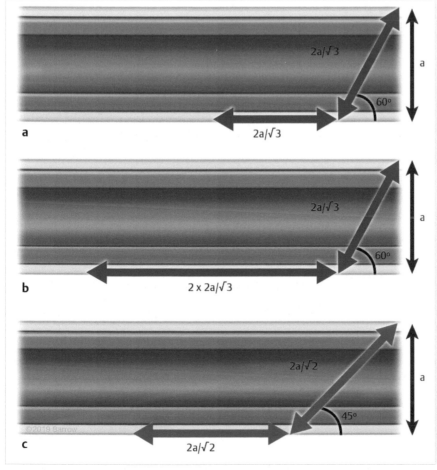

Fig. 3.32 Patterns and geometry of the donor vessel orifice in fish-mouth technique. **(a)** The geometry of the fish-mouth opening when the vessel end is cut obliquely at 60 degrees, and the side wall is incised to the same length as the oblique cut. **(b)** The same 60-degree oblique cut but with the side wall incised twice as long as a typical oblique cut. **(c)**. The oblique cut is made at a sharper angle (45-degree angle is shown) and with the side cut the same length as the length of the oblique vessel end cut. The formulas are given to show the cut distances relative to the vessel diameter (a).

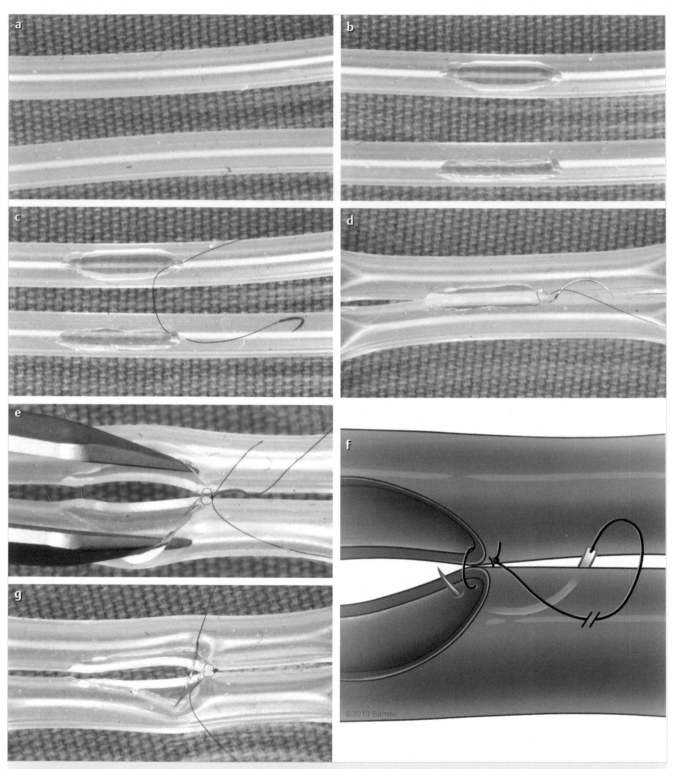

Fig. 3.33 Stepwise technique for side-to-side anastomosis. **(a)** Two vessels are aligned parallel to each other. **(b)** After temporary clips (*not shown*) are placed, two equal size openings are created. A longitudinal cut is sufficient in small caliber vessels, but in vessels larger than 1 mm in diameter and in rigid silicone tubes, oval openings are required for optimal approximation. **(c)** The first suture is placed on the right side of the vessels to be anastomosed. **(d)** As the first suture is tightened, the two vessels are pulled closer together. **(e)** Photograph and **(f)** illustration showing an important step: the needle is passed from the right side, in-between the two vessels, outside of the anastomosis and punctured back wall of the lower vessel from outside in. **(g)** Next, the running suture is started on the back wall from the inside, moving from right to left. (*Continued*)

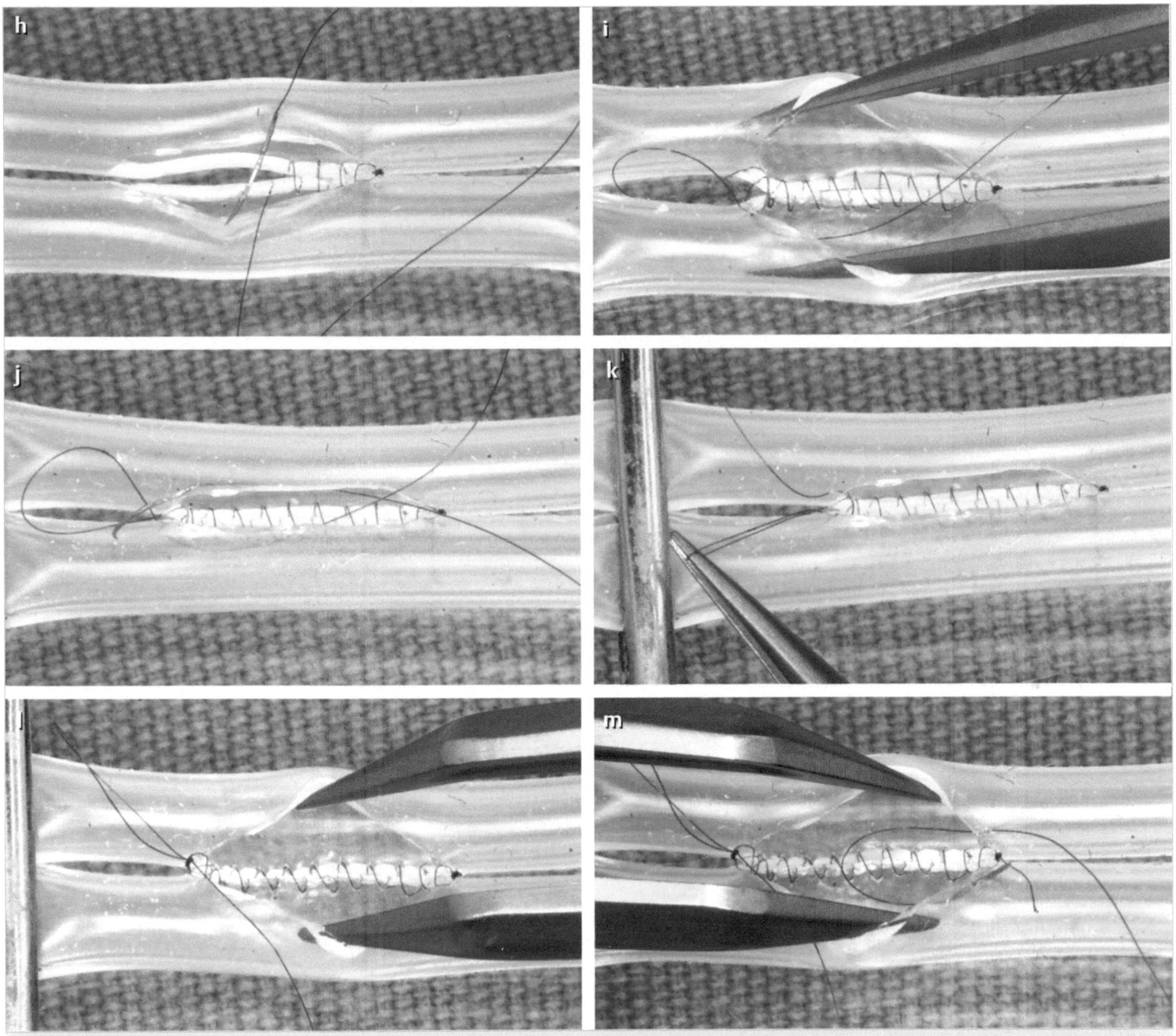

Fig. 3.33 (*Continued*) **(h)** Running suture in this direction leaves enough free space inside the anastomosis for the left-hand instrument to apply counterpressure. **(i)** A loose outside loop is left free at the left corner of the anastomosis in preparation for the securing knot, while the needle exits inside the vessel. **(j)** Next, the needle is passed from the inside to the outside. **(k)** The previously created loop and the suture with the needle are facing outside at the left corner. **(l)** The running suture on the back wall should be tightened now and fixed with the securing knot. The suture ends are left uncut. **(m)** Now we start a running suture on the front wall, again in a right-to-left direction, which is more comfortable for suturing if the surgeon is right handed. (*Continued*)

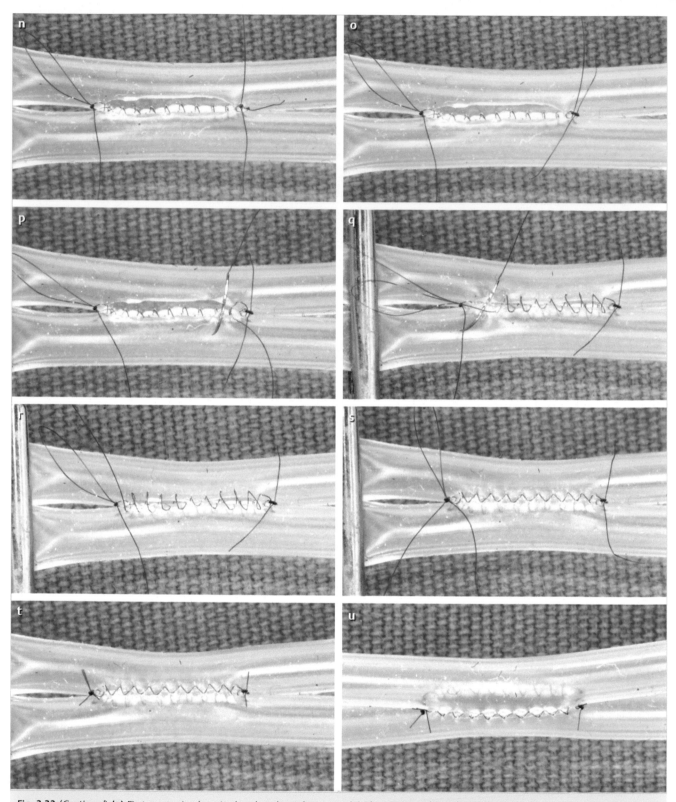

Fig. 3.33 (*Continued*) **(n)** First, a securing knot is placed at the right corner. **(o)** This suture is also tightened with the back wall suture. **(p)** Running suture is placed in the outside-in then inside-out fashion on the joining edges using single needle passes. **(q)** There is no need to leave an outside loop, as this upper suture can be tightened to the previously left end of the back wall suture. **(r)** The front wall suture end is aligned with the end tail of the back wall suture. **(s)** Running suture loops are tightened, and the front wall suture is secured with the back wall suture at the left corner of anastomosis. **(t)** The suture ends are trimmed. **(u)** Clips are released, and the anastomosis is rotated to show the orifice through the transparent wall. (*Continued*)

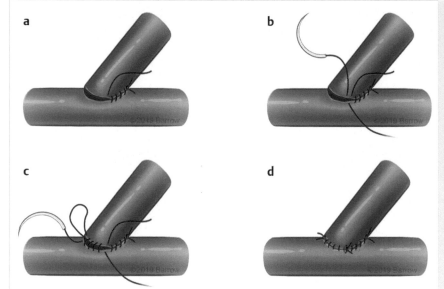

Fig. 3.34 Repair of a ruptured running suture. **(a)** Example of a continuous suture that ruptured at the middle of the run. **(b)** The new suture started at the same point, but on the opposite side of the opening. **(c)** The new suture is finished and secured at the anastomosis toe. **(d)** The ends of the first and second sutures are tied together at the middle to secure the anastomosis.

Sidebar

Main objectives for learning the skills of microvascular suturing:
1. To minimize the physiological tremor in maximal magnification of the microscope
2. To develop psychological stability against nervousness
3. To learn slow but exact manipulating patterns
4. To learn how to grasp the vessel by the periadventitial sheath and to fixate the recipient artery
5. To learn how to puncture all three layers of the vessel wall using the counter-press method
6. To master suturing with both the left and the right hands

References

[1] Fargen KM, Turner RD, Spiotta AM. Factors that affect physiologic tremor and dexterity during surgery: a primer for neurosurgeons. World Neurosurg; 86: 384–389

[2] World Anti-Doping Agency. P2. Beta-blockers. 2016. Available at: https://www .wada-ama.org/en/content/what-is-prohibited/prohibited-in-particular-sports /beta-blockers. Accessed December 3, 2019

[3] Elman MJ, Sugar J, Fiscella R, et al. The effect of propranolol versus placebo on resident surgical performance. Trans Am Ophthalmol Soc; 96:283–291, discussion 291–294

[4] Pointdujour R, Ahmad H, Liu M, Smith E, Lazzaro D. β-blockade affects simulator scores. Ophthalmology; 118(9):1893–1893.e3

[5] Humayun MU, Rader RS, Pieramici DJ, Awh CC, de Juan E , Jr. Quantitative measurement of the effects of caffeine and propranolol on surgeon hand tremor. Arch Ophthalmol; 115(3):371–374

[6] Hashimoto N, Kikuta K. Excellent basic cerebrovascular surgical skills. [in Japanese]. Med Publ (Oulu)

[7] Belykh E, Byvaltsev V. Off-the-job microsurgical training on dry models: Siberian experience. World Neurosurg; 82(1–2):20–24

[8] LifeLike BioTissue's Microvessels. Available at: http://lifelikebiotissue.com /shop/obgyn-urology/microvessels. Accessed December 3, 2019.

[9] Mutoh T, Ishikawa T, Ono H, Yasui N. A new polyvinyl alcohol hydrogel vascular model (KEZLEX) for microvascular anastomosis training. Surg Neurol Int; 1:74

[10] Inoue T, Tsutsumi K, Adachi S, Tanaka S, Saito K, Kunii N. Effectiveness of suturing training with 10–0 nylon under fixed and maximum magnification (x 20) using desk type microscope. Surg Neurol; 66(2):183–187

[11] Matsumura N, Hayashi N, Hamada H, Shibata T, Horie Y, Endo S. A newly designed training tool for microvascular anastomosis techniques: microvascular practice card. Surg Neurol; 71(5):616–620

[12] Senior MA, Southern SJ, Majumder S. Microvascular simulator—a device for micro-anastomosis training. Ann R Coll Surg Engl; 83(5):358–360

[13] Cobbett J. Small vessel anastomosis. A comparison of suture techniques. Br J Plast Surg; 20(1):16–20

[14] MacDonald JD. Learning to perform microvascular anastomosis. Skull Base; 15(3):229–240

[15] Loth F, Fischer PF, Bassiouny HS. Blood flow in end-to-side anastomoses. Annu Rev Fluid Mech; 40:367–393

[16] Yaşargil M. Microsurgery: Applied to Neurosurgery. Stuttgart: Thieme; 2006

[17] Chen L, Chiu DT. Spiral interrupted suturing technique for microvascular anastomosis: a comparative study. Microsurgery. 1986;7:72-78.

[18] Rennert RC, Strickland BA, Radwanski RE, et al. Running-to-interrupted microsuture technique for vascular bypass. Oper neurosurg (Hagerstown). 2018;15:412-417.

4 Day 3: Wet-Laboratory Microsurgical Training: Basic Principles for Working with Laboratory Animals

Evgenii Belykh and Nikolay L. Martirosyan

Abstract

Microneurosurgical training using laboratory animals is often considered as a final preparatory step before performing microvascular anastomosis on a patient. Such training should begin with a training session on the use and care of laboratory animals according to the guidelines of the particular institution. This chapter does not replace such institutional training but is intended to reinforce and briefly summarize critical points about laboratory safety, animal care, animal handling, anesthesia, and general surgical approaches. It also provides summarized information that would be of use in each wet-laboratory training session.

Keywords: anesthesia, animal care, ethics, microneurosurgical training, rat, surgical approach, wet-laboratory training

4.1 Basic Principles of Working with Laboratory Animals

To begin training, one must first become familiar with the rules of the laboratory and with handling laboratory animals. One's attitude toward laboratory animals must be as humane and respectful as it is to humans in acknowledgment of the sacrifice made.

In order to work with laboratory animals, an application for the work should be approved by an ethics committee at the institution. In many countries, there is a formal body (e.g., an institutional animal care and use committee) that supervises such work and ensures that it adheres to international standards. The researcher takes responsibility to ensure that the care of the animals is exemplary and, if necessary, may be obligated to take care of the animals personally, including feeding, watering, anaesthetizing during pain or distress, and promptly performing euthanasia, if needed.

Considering the necessity of information about handling laboratory animals and the relatively rare literature on this topic, we decided to provide essential principles that everyone who undergoes microsurgical training should know.

4.2 The Three "R" Principles

In most countries, researchers are guided by the three "R" principles for humane treatment of research animals that were proposed by William Moy Stratton Russell and Rex Leonard Burch in 1959.[1] These principles are referred to as reduction, refinement, and replacement. *Reduction* refers to methods that enable researchers to obtain comparable levels of information from fewer animals or to obtain more information from the same number of animals; *refinement* refers to methods that alleviate or minimize potential pain, suffering, or distress and enhance welfare for the animals used; and *replacement* is the practice of preferring to use nonanimal methods over animal methods whenever it is possible to achieve the same scientific aim.

4.3 Symptoms of Pain and Distress in Laboratory Animals

When working with laboratory animals, it is important to be able to recognize the signs of pain and distress that they may exhibit. *Pain* is defined as an unpleasant sensory and emotional experience associated with potential or actual tissue damage, or described in terms of such damage (from the International Association for the Study of Pain). *Distress* is defined as the biological responses that an animal exhibits in an attempt to cope with a threat to its homeostasis.[2] Signs of pain and distress in laboratory animals are presented in ▶ Table 4.1 and ▶ Fig. 4.1.

4.4 Anesthesia

Appropriate pain relief and sedation, as well as proper care of laboratory animals, are the responsibility of the researcher. There are two primary ways to induce anesthesia: injection and inhalation. Injection can be performed via intravenous, intraperitoneal, or intramuscular (▶ Fig. 4.2) routes.

The mode of anesthesia is usually chosen based on the availability of a certain drug and the peculiarities of the study being undertaken. A variety of injectable pharmaceuticals useful for the narcosis of laboratory rats is presented in ▶ Table 4.2.[3,4,5,6,7,8,9] Metabolism is higher in rodents than in humans, and drugs are therefore metabolized and excreted faster. Thus, dosages for anesthetics differ significantly from those for humans. Many substances are narcotics and require special permission and conditions for their storage and use.

For rat anesthesia during microsurgical training, we prefer using a xylazine/ketamine cocktail. The recommended combination is 8 mL of 100 mg/mL ketamine + 1 mL of 100 mg/mL xylazine + 1 mL of sterile isotonic saline, resulting in 10 mL total cocktail. The dosage of 0.1 mL per 100 g intramuscular injection delivers 10 mg/kg xylazine and 80 mg/kg ketamine.

Laboratory animals are small in size, so the volume of injected solution is small (▶ Table 4.3). For aqueous solutions, intramuscular injection sites should be rotated. For nonaqueous solutions, not more than two intramuscular injection sites and not more than three subcutaneous injection sites should be used per day.[10] Intraperitoneal injections should be infrequent in survival experiments due to the risk of peritonitis.

4.5 Blood Loss

In the case of blood loss during surgery or when taking blood for analysis, one should follow the parameters described in ▶ Table 4.4. After a loss of 7.5% of total circulating blood

Table 4.1 Potential signs associated with pain or distress in laboratory animals

Symptom	Laboratory animals		
	Mice	Rats	Rabbits
Decreased food and water consumption	+	+	+
Weight loss	+	+	+
Self-imposed isolation/hiding	+	+	+
Self-mutilation, gnawing at limbs	+	+	+
Rapid breathing	+	+	+
Opened-mouth breathing	+	+	+
Abdominal breathing	+	+	+
Grinding teeth	–	+	+
Biting/growling/aggression	–	+	+
Increased/decreased movement	+	+	+
Unkempt appearance (erected, matted, or dull coat)	+	+	+
Abnormal posture/positioning (e.g., head-pressing, hunched back)	+	+	+
Restless sleep	–	–	+
Tearing (including porphyrin staining), lack of blinking reflex	–	+	+
Dilated pupils	–	–	+
Muscle rigidity, lack of muscle tone	+	+	+
Dehydration/skin tenting/sunken eyes	+	+	+
Twitching, trembling, tremor	+	+	+
Vocalization (rare)	+	+	+
Redness or swelling around surgical site	+	+	+
Increased salivation	–	–	+

Source: Adapted from Office of Animal Care and Use: Guidelines for Pain and Distress in Laboratory Animals: Responsibilities, Recognition and Alleviation. Bethesda, MD: Office of Animal Care and Use, National Institutes of Health, 2015. Available at: https://oacu.oir.nih.gov/animal-research-advisory-committee-guidelines.

volume, an animal will need 1 week for recovery, and they need 2 weeks of recovery time after a 10% blood loss.[10]

4.6 Euthanasia

A humane ending for each experiment should be planned. Experiments with laboratory animals should be completed with euthanasia. According to the American Veterinary Medical Association, methods of euthanasia are considered as either *acceptable*, *conditionally acceptable* (requires institutional animal care and use committee approval of scientific justification), or *unacceptable*.[11]

4.6.1 Acceptable Methods of Euthanasia

The following methods of euthanasia are considered acceptable:
- Barbiturates (most species)
- Carbon dioxide—bottled gas only (most species)
- Inhalant anesthetics (most species)
- Microwave (commercial grade) irradiation (mice and rats)
- Tricaine methanesulfonate (abbreviation: TMS or MS-222; fish, amphibians)
- Benzocaine hydrochloride (fish, amphibians)

- Captive penetrating bolt (horse, ruminant, swine)
- Ether and carbon monoxide are acceptable for many species, but they are relatively dangerous to personnel.

Conditionally Acceptable Methods of Euthanasia

The following methods of euthanasia are considered conditionally acceptable:
- Cervical dislocation (birds, small rodents, and rabbits)
- Decapitation (birds, rodents, some other species)
- Pithing (some ectotherms)
- Various pharmacological and physical methods

Unacceptable Methods of Euthanasia

The following methods of euthanasia are *not* considered acceptable, and should not be used:
- Chloral hydrate, chloroform, and cyanide
- Decompression
- Neuromuscular blockers
- Various pharmacological and physical methods
- Dry ice-generated carbon dioxide

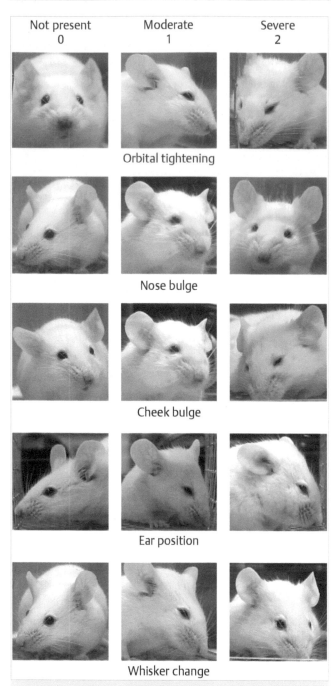

Not present 0	Moderate 1	Severe 2

Orbital tightening

Nose bulge

Cheek bulge

Ear position

Whisker change

Fig. 4.1 Coding of facial expressions of pain in the laboratory mouse from the mouse grimace scale could be used to detect and understand the animal pain and distress. The grimaces are subjectively graded from 0 (not present) to 2 (severe) to make a global pain/no pain assessment. (Reproduced with permission from Langford DJ, Bailey AL, Chanda ML, et al. Coding of facial expressions of pain in the laboratory mouse. Nat Methods. 2010;7:447–449.)

4.7 Hazards in Animal Research

Working with animals in the laboratory carries the following dangers:
- Allergies from urine, dandruff, hair, etc.
- Bites from rats and mice, kicks from rabbits, scratches
- Infectious diseases (e.g., zoonoses, hantavirus, and lymphocytic choriomeningitis virus)
- Spreading of disease among the laboratory animals, which is a reason for maintaining a strict isolation regimen in the laboratory, including the use of special clothing or gowns, changing shoes upon entering, and limiting access to the animals to essential staff only
- Needle sticks (which may involve the injection of toxic substances, pathogens, or tumor cells)
- Inhalation of poisonous substances (e.g., formalin, which is a carcinogen)

One should follow strict rules for working with laboratory animals. Clean, protective clothing must be worn, including a laboratory coat, cap, mask, gloves, and footwear. One should avoid touching one's face and eyes in the laboratory. Special attention should be taken when handling needles. Handling animals should be done with delicacy and with care, using restrictive devices or sedation, as needed. The animal room must have good ventilation, especially when working with inhalational anesthetics and formalin. Doors should be kept closed to limit access to the animal room. After exiting the laboratory, one should wash hands and face thoroughly with disinfectant soap and water.

4.8 Microneurosurgical Training in a Wet Laboratory

Microneurosurgery training with biological materials, such as live animals, also called wet-laboratory training, allows the trainee to obtain the skills of dissecting biological tissue and creating anastomoses. Training with laboratory animals allows a unique opportunity to assess the long-term patency of anastomoses. This type of training is considered to be the most efficient, but it also demands more equipment.

The basic exercises for training in a wet laboratory for the development of skills needed in neurosurgery practice are described in the following chapters. Such exercises can be used not only to develop microneurosurgical skills but also to support them during one's whole neurosurgical career.[12]

This chapter will serve as a reference guide for the approach to a particular anatomical region of a rat, so subsequent chapters will not repeat this information, but will instead concentrate on the technical aspects of anastomosis and other microsurgical techniques.

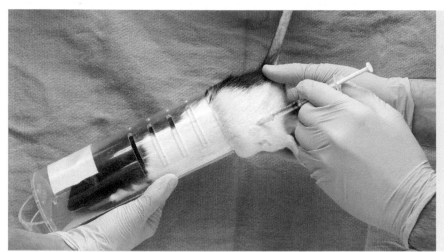

Fig. 4.2 Rat anesthesia by intramuscular drug injection. Take rat by the tail and put it into the restriction device for easy and safe injection of drugs into the animal's thigh muscles.

Table 4.2 Injectable anesthetics and application doses for rats

Drug	Trade names	Dose	Effect	Duration, minute	Sleep, minute	Reference
Ketamine + acepromazine		30–75 mg/kg + 2.5–3 mg/kg IM or IP	Light anesthesia	20–30	120	3,5
Ketamine/diazepam	Valium	40–80 mg/kg + 5–10 mg/kg IP	Light anesthesia	20–30	120	3,5
Ketamine + dexmedetomidine	Dexdomitor	60–80 mg/kg + 0.1–0.25 mg/kg IP	Surgical anesthesia, dexmedetomidine should not be re-dosed	20–30	120–240	3,4
Ketamine + midazolam	Versed	60–80 mg/kg + 5 mg/kg IP	Light anesthesia	20–30	120	3,5
Ketamine + xylazine	Rompun	50–100 mg/kg + 5–10 mg/kg IP or IM	Surgical anesthesia, xylazine should not be re-dosed	20–30	120–240	3,7
Methohexital 1% solution	Brevital	7–15 mg/kg IV	Light anesthesia	5	10	6
Pentobarbital	Nembutal	30–60 mg/kg IP	Light anesthesia	15–60	120–240	3,7,8
Propofol	Diprivan, Rapinovet	7.5–10 mg/kg IV (induction); 44–55 mg/kg/h (maintenance)	Surgical anesthesia	5	10	3,6
Thiopental	Pentothal	30 mg/kg IV; 50 mg/kg IP	Surgical anesthesia	10	15	3,5
Tiletamine/zolazepam	Telazol	20–40 mg/kg IP or 20 mg/kg IM	Light anesthesia	15–25	60–120	9
Urethane[a]		1,000 mg/kg IP	Surgical anesthesia	360–480	60–120	3

Abbreviations: IM, intramuscular; IP, intraperitoneal; IV, intravenous.
[a]Tumor inducer; use only in nonrecovery experiments.

Table 4.3 Administration volumes considered good practice (and possible maximal dose volumes)

Species	Route, volumes, mL/kg[a]					
	Oral	SC	IP	IM	IV (bolus)	IV (slow injection)
Mice	10 (50)	10 (40)	20 (80)	0.05[b] (0.1)[b]	5	(25)
Rat	10 (40)	5 (10)	10 (20)	0.1[b] (0.2)[b]	5	(20)
Rabbits	10 (15)	1 (2)	5 (20)	0.25 (0.5)	2	(10)

Abbreviations: IM, intramuscular; IP, intraperitoneal; IV, intravenous; SC, subcutaneous.
[a]Numbers in parentheses represent possible maximal dose volumes.
[b]mL/site
Source: Adapted from Diehl et al.[10]

Table 4.4 Total blood volumes and recommended maximum blood sample volumes

Species (body weight)	Total blood volume, mL	Blood loss volume, mL			
		7.5%	10%	15%	20%
Mice (25 g)	1.8	0.1	0.2	0.3	0.4
Rat (250 g)	16	1.2	1.6	2.4	3.2
Rabbits (4 kg)	224	17	22	34	45
Source: Adapted from Diehl et al.[10]					

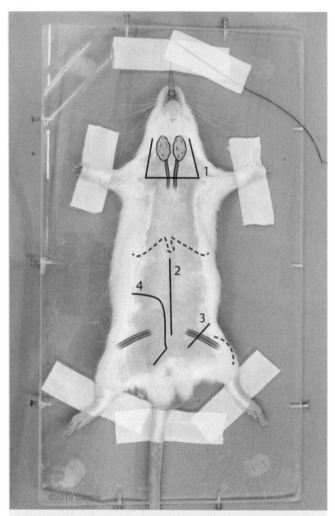

Fig. 4.3 Laboratory rat immobilized before procedure. Incision sites are marked in black. **1**, approach to the carotid arteries (using a flap incision); **2**, approach to the abdominal cavity (via a midline laparotomy); **3 and 4**, approaches to the femoral vessels. The knee (*purple dashed line*) serves as a landmark for the location of the femoral artery and vein (*red and blue lines*). The femoral vascular bundle exits from the inguinal ligament and runs laterally in the direction slightly inferior to the knee joint. The inferior costal edge is marked with the *dark blue dashed line*. The submandibular salivary glands are shown in an artist's overlay in *pink*.

After induction of anesthesia, the rat is placed on a tray (▶ Fig. 4.3). Its extremities are fixed in position with tape or rubber bands. The animal's hair is removed from the surgical site with the help of a scalpel, razor blade, or depilatory cream. Cut hairs should be thoroughly removed with a generous amount of tape so that they do not distract the trainee during the microsurgical steps. Warming tools, such as infrared lamps or heated pads, should be used if necessary to keep the animal normothermic during long training sessions, especially in survival experiments. Rats will almost certainly require additional anesthesia after about 1 to 2 hours of training, so the anesthetic dose should be prepared ahead of time.

4.8.1 Approach to the Femoral Neurovascular Bundle

To approach the femoral neurovascular bundle, a skin incision is made in the iliac region, either in a linear fashion parallel to the vessel bundle, or perpendicular to the vessel bundle, or as a flap (▶ Fig. 4.3). Under the skin, between the trunk muscles and the femoral muscles, there is a pad of adipose tissue containing the epigastric artery and vein; this adipose tissue should be reflected superiorly. Later, this tissue flap can be used for covering the anastomosis to stop the bleeding. The adipose pad can be dissected circularly clockwise starting at 2 o'clock and ending at 11 o'clock (when approaching the left side) and then turned up. This method of dissection allows for opening of the neurovascular bundle between the quadriceps and popliteal muscles and also saves the vascularized adipose flap. Medially located muscles of the abdominal wall should be retracted medially with the custom retractors until the inguinal ligament can be visualized. This ligament is a thick white band that serves as a landmark for the proximal border of the dissection. Retractors are then positioned appropriately to create a wide operative field for dissection.

The microscope is set to low magnification for dissection of the vessels. The dark-colored femoral vein is more noticeable than the artery. The artery may be differentiated from the vein by its size, which is smaller in diameter (1.0–0.8 mm) than the vein, and by its color, which is lighter than the vein due to the thicker layer of the adventitia, by its visible pulsation, and by its position, as it usually runs deep to the vein. The thin, semitransparent femoral nerve, containing 3 to 5 bundles, is located near the artery. This nerve requires very careful dissection. The vein, artery, and nerve should be dissected from the surrounding tissues, so that about 1 cm of vessel length is dissected free. Usually, dissection of the vessel segment for anastomosis can be done proximal to the epigastric vessel bundle, encountered at the beginning of the approach, where the vessel diameter is larger compared to the vessel segment distal to the epigastric branch.

Working in a direction from proximal to distal, lift the adventitia covering the neurovascular bundle with microsurgery forceps (in the left hand) and dissect the connective tissue sharply from the vessels with the microsurgery scissors (in the right hand). The basic technique of vessel dissection from the surrounding tissues is similar to almost all vessels, including dissection of the femoral artery and vein in the rat, dissection of the superficial temporal artery in humans and, in part, dissection of cortical cerebral vessels in humans (▶ Fig. 4.4).

Approximately at the center of the femoral approach, a small arterial branch, also known as Murphey's artery, arises from the back wall of the femoral artery (▶ Fig. 4.5). This branch should be ligated with 10–0 suture to allow mobility of the femoral artery. Avulsion of this artery could create significant bleeding and require subsequent repair. The importance of a clean and bloodless operative field cannot be overestimated during creation of the anastomosis. The surface of the approach should be constantly moistened with heparinized isotonic

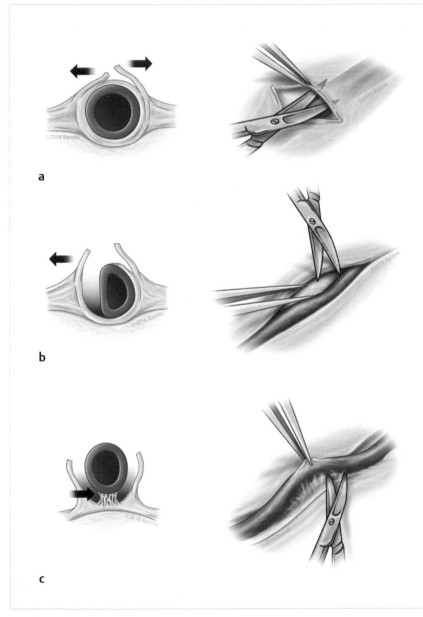

Fig. 4.4 Basic technique for dissecting a vessel out of its connective tissue sheath. A short opening is made in the connective tissue covering the vessel. **(a)** Then, the sheath is bluntly dissected out from the top wall of the artery and incised along the artery. **(b)** Dissect one side of the artery, then repeat for the opposite side. **(c)** Finally, gently lift the artery, holding it by the periadventitial tissues, and dissect the bottom adhesions of the artery with the microsurgical scissors.

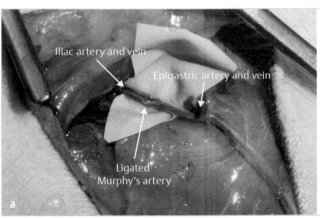

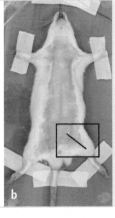

Fig. 4.5 Exposure of the femoral vessels. **(a)** The left femoral artery and vein are dissected proximal to the epigastric vascular bundle. **(b)** Anatomical location and orientation of the approach.

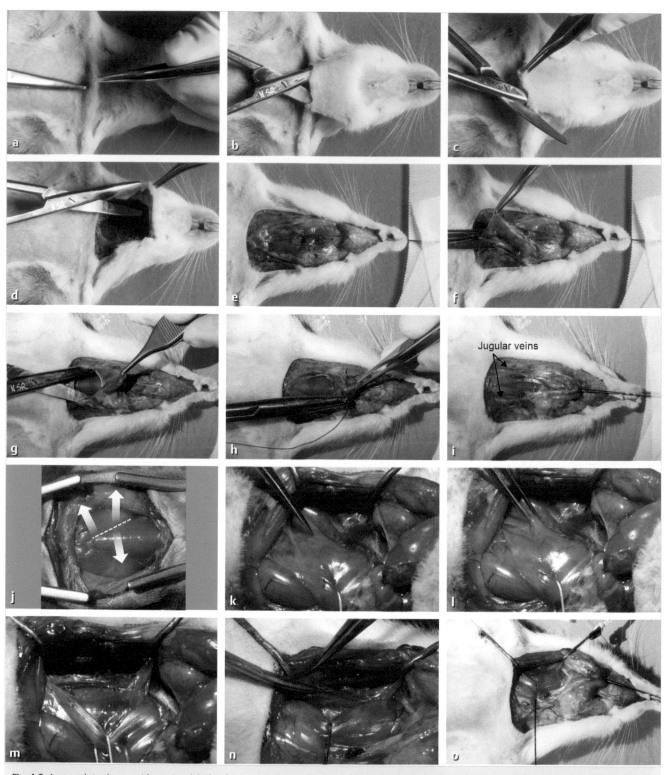

Fig. 4.6 Approach to the carotid arteries. **(a)** The skin is incised over the sternum and **(b)** scissors are used to dissect subcutaneously. Vertical cuts are made on the left **(c)** and right **(d)** sides creating a cutaneous flap. **(e)** The flap is rotated upward and fixed with a suture. **(f)** The fascia is dissected starting from the sternum. **(g)** The fascia is incised along the jugular veins, taking care not to injure the vessels. The submandibular glands are easily identified and should be retracted rostrally. **(h)** The fascial flap is rotated upward and fixed with a suture. **(i)** The jugular veins can be identified and dissected at this step or at a later stage. **(j)** The muscles are retracted to the sides with a custom retractor. **(k)** The oblique muscle bundle covering the carotid arteries is exposed, **(l)** dissected bluntly, and **(m)** retracted laterally with two retractors. **(n)** The carotid sheath is opened with scissors. **(o)** The final exposure containing the vagus nerve and carotid artery is shown.

solution to prevent tissues from drying out under the light of the microscope. Small gauze tissues or cotton rounds and sticks are used to remove blood and excess fluid. Papaverine solution can be applied locally to prevent vasospasm. When the vessels have been dissected free from the surrounding tissue, they are ready to be used in the exercises.

4.8.2 Approach to the Neck Vessels

Depending on the goal of the experiment, either a linear incision or a curved cutaneous incision can be performed. A linear incision should be chosen for survival experiments, whereas a large cutaneous flap can be used for termination experiments, as it allows more working space, easy access to the anatomy, and fewer hairs near the anastomosis. The main steps of carotid exposure are presented in ▶ Fig. 4.6. One should pay attention while dissecting the cervical fascia, as it contains many veins and small arteries, including the jugular vein, which may look like avascular tissue when it is surgically put under tension during dissection. A careless tear or cut in this vessel could create significant bleeding. After exposing the neck muscles, the sternocleidomastoid muscle, which runs obliquely, should be retracted laterally. If mobilization of this muscle is needed for

adequate exposure, care should be taken to coagulate or ligate its feeding vascular bundle. After retraction of the sternocleidomastoid and midline muscles apart, the last thin muscle covering the carotid artery is exposed. This muscle may be retracted laterally or cut after its vascular supply has been identified and ligated or coagulated.

The carotid artery can be seen as a pulsating vessel contained in the white bundle of the vagus nerve. Care should be taken to dissect the artery proximally and distally, to prevent injury to the vagus nerve, as injuring the vagus nerve may affect animal survival.

4.8.3 Midline Laparotomy

Midline laparotomy is an extensive invasive approach and should preferably be performed last if multiple approaches are undertaken. This approach is relatively straightforward. The major steps of midline laparotomy are presented in ▶ Fig. 4.7. Special caution and aseptic conditions are required for survival experiments, while for termination procedures, less care is necessary. The exposed content of the abdominal cavity should be continuously moistened to prevent it from drying out. The animal's intestines are usually taken out, retracted to the right and kept in moistened surgical gauze. The aorta and vena cava are

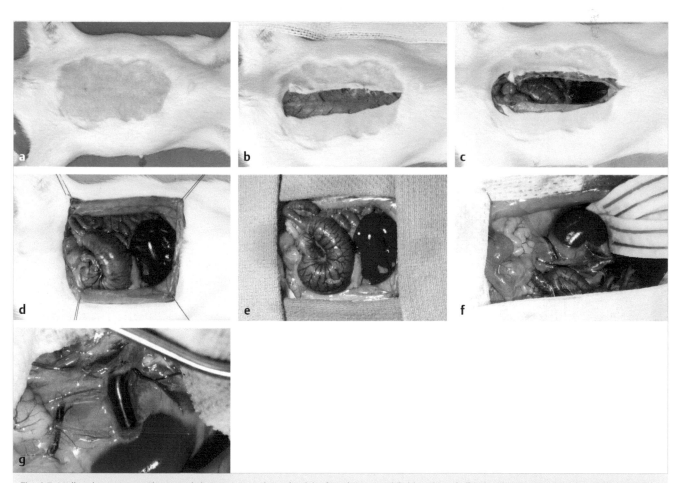

Fig. 4.7 Midline laparotomy. The rostral direction is to the right. **(a)** After the surgical field is shaved, **(b)** the skin is incised at the midline. **(c)** The peritoneum is then opened with scissors beginning near the xyphoid process and proceeding caudally, and **(d)** the wound edges are retracted to the sides with stay sutures. **(e)** The surgical field is draped. **(f)** The intestines are then moved aside and covered with moistened surgical gauze, exposing the right kidney, pulsating aorta, and inferior vena cava. The liver may also be retracted upwards with wet cottonoids. **(g)** The left kidney is exposed, and the renal vein is visible at the center of the exposure.

frequently hidden beneath a layer of adipose tissue, but can be easily recognized by its pulsation. The aorta lies to the left and behind the vena cava, and it is significantly smaller and brighter than the vena cava.

Knowledge of the rat anatomy and experimentation with various approaches allows safe and fast access in order to save time for the actual anastomosis training. However, training in gentle tissue handling during dissection of delicate animal tissues as a preparatory step should not be underestimated. Preparation of a bloodless, clean, hydrated (not dried out!), and unobstructed operative field is one of the key factors for successful anastomosis.

References

[1] Russell WMS, Burch RL. The Principles of Humane Experimental Technique. London: Methuen; 1959

[2] Carstens E, Moberg GP. Recognizing pain and distress in laboratory animals. ILAR J; 41(2):62–71

[3] Flecknell PA. Laboratory Animal Anesthesia. 3rd ed. London: Academic Press; 2009

[4] Boston University Research Support. Compliance. Available at: http://www.bu.edu/researchsupport/compliance/. Accessed March 23, 2018

[5] University of California, San Diego, Animal Care Program. Tranquilizers, analgesics and anesthetics for use in rodents & lagomorphs. 2013. Available at: http://blink.ucsd.edu/_files/sponsor-tab/iacuc/Rodent_Rabbit_Anesthesia.pdf. Accessed December 3, 2019

[6] West Virginia University Institutional Care and Use Committee. WVU IACUC Approved Guidelines: Anesthesia and Analgesia in Rats. SOP no. 11–012: West Virginia University; 2011

[7] Fish RE, Brown MJ, Danneman PJ, Karas AZ. Anesthesia and Analgesia in Laboratory Animals. 2nd ed. New York, NY: Academic Press; 2008

[8] Carpenter JW. Exotic Animal Formulary. 3rd ed. St. Louis, MO: Elsevier Saunders; 2005

[9] Hillyer EV, Quesenberry KE. Ferrets, Rabbits, and Rodents: Clinical Medicine and Surgery. 1st ed. New York, NY: W.B. Saunders; 1997

[10] Diehl KH, Hull R, Morton D, et al. European Federation of Pharmaceutical Industries Association and European Centre for the Validation of Alternative Methods. A good practice guide to the administration of substances and removal of blood, including routes and volumes. J Appl Toxicol; 21(1):15–23

[11] American Veterinary Medical Association. AVMA Guidelines for the Euthanasia of Animals: 2013 Edition. 2013. Available at: https://www.avma.org/KB/Policies/Documents/euthanasia.pdf. Accessed December 3, 2019

[12] Ryuhei K, Ken-ichiro K. Off-the-job Neurosurgical training System at University of Fukui: lifelong education for neurosurgeons. Jpn J Neurosurg.; 19(5):388–394

5 Day 4: Exercise Set 1: Basic Arterial Anastomoses

Evgenii Belykh and Nikolay L. Martirosyan

Abstract

In this chapter, we describe techniques for suturing basic vascular microanastomoses on biological tissues and introduce principles of microvascular suturing. We describe continuous and interrupted sutures in end-to-side anastomosis, end-to-end anastomosis, and side-to-side anastomosis.

Keywords: carotid artery, end-to-end anastomosis, end-to-side anastomosis, femoral artery, laboratory animals, rat, side-to-side anastomosis

5.1 Vascular Suturing

The walls of small arteries consist of three layers: the intima, which faces the lumen; the media; and the adventitia, which is the outermost layer. The intima consists of a monolayer of endothelial cells and internal elastic lamina. Smooth muscle cell proliferation and atheromatous plaques are usually observed in intima of aged patients. The media occupies up to 80% of the thickness of the vascular wall and, depending on the order of segments of arteries, includes varied layers of smooth muscle cells, a small amount of elastic fibers, and a collagen framework. In small terminal branches of cerebral vessels, the elastic fibers of the media are usually absent, and the media consists mostly of reticulin fibers and smooth muscle cells. Of the three layers, the media provides the most strength for the vascular suture because of its pronounced collagen network.[1] The adventitia has the highest thrombogenic properties.

There are several basic requirements for microvascular sutures. Correctly placed sutures will:
- Permit no major leakage from the vessel
- Allow precise coaptation of the intima
- Be durable
- Cause no narrowing of the lumen
- Leave no sutures or adventitia in the lumen

The main requirement for a vascular suture is that it is tight enough to prevent leaks. The choice of appropriate needles and sutures is one of the most important factors for successful vascular suturing. Most microsurgical needles are curved, although straight needles are sometimes used for end-to-end microanastomosis. Inexpensive, nonsterile sutures can be chosen for training; however, only special vascular needles should be used for surgery. The following sizes of sutures are usually used: 11–0 for a vessel diameter of less than 1 mm, 10–0 for a vessel diameter of 1 mm, 9–0 for a vessel diameter of 2 mm, and 8–0 and larger for a vessel diameter of more than 2 mm. The carotid artery is sutured with 6–0 sutures.

In anastomosis of two vessels of unequal sizes, approximation of the vessel walls should be performed only within their natural elasticity by slight stretching. Overstretching of the vessel wall can damage the intima or the entire wall and can result in bleeding or thrombosis during or after the surgery.

Weakness of the vascular wall at the anastomosis may also result in aneurysm formation.

The suturing must be precise, and the connection of intimal layers is very important in vascular suturing. The muscular membrane or the adventitial cover must not get into the lumen of sutured vessels; otherwise, they may cause thrombosis and failure of the anastomosis.

When all the knots on one side have been formed, the vessels should be turned to check the quality of the sutures from inside. The common mistakes are shown in ▶ Fig. 5.1.

5.2 Exercise: End-to-End Anastomosis on Rat Carotid Arteries

This exercise simulates rare neurosurgical situations where end-to-end anastomosis is needed, primarily for in situ intracranial reconstructions. Performing end-to-end anastomosis is a relatively straightforward task (▶ Fig. 5.2, Video 5.1). However, there are several critical nuances that can make suturing either easy and successful or difficult and unsuccessful.

To begin, you should prepare and dissect a clean and wide operative field with sufficient length of vessel available. Next, apply the clip approximator in either of the two ways. The first and most common method is to place it horizontally for the front wall exposure and then to rotate it 180 degrees for the back wall exposure. This procedure can be used if the vessel length allows for this degree of axial rotation. The second method is to apply the clip approximator vertically, then rotate it 90 degrees in one direction for front wall exposure, and then 90 degrees in the other direction for back wall exposure. This method can be used for short vessels that do not allow much axial rotation. If no rotation is possible, which is relatively common, then the back wall can be sutured from the inside, like in a side-to-side anastomosis, or you can use a single stay suture technique.

Adventitia should be cleaned from the vessel ends for a distance that allows for safe and convenient vessel end approximation and for choice of the needle puncture site, usually about half the diameter of the vessel. Arteries will be in a contracted state at this step, so you may want to dilate them with a dilator or forceps, which will help you to make even spaces between the sutures later. Stay sutures are commonly used in microsurgical practice for end-to-end anastomosis because they help to hold the vessel lumen open. When used, stay sutures are placed in the free ends of the arteries and are secured in slits of a silicon dam or on an approximator. However, in neurosurgery, arteries are usually not as small, so this step can be omitted. In addition, an approximator does not always fit in the space available in operative approaches within the brain, so they are less likely to be used in actual surgery.

There are three common strategies for beginning interrupted vascular suturing with stay sutures: two stay sutures may be

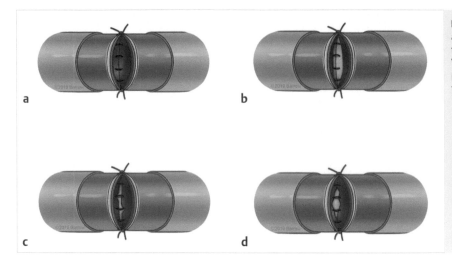

Fig. 5.1 Possible defects in performing anastomosis. **(a)** Loose knots (the sutures are in the lumen of the vessel). **(b)** Peeled off intima. **(c)** Vessel wall cut by the sutures and with the intima peeled off. **(d)** The adventitia is in the lumen of the vessel.

placed 180 degrees apart[2]; two stay sutures may be placed 120 degrees apart[3]; or one stay suture may be placed in the back wall and suturing continued from both sides.[4]

While suturing, gently grab the vessel wall by the remaining adventitia with forceps and avoid applying pressure to the media and intima. Use the counter-press technique for passing the needle. For end-to-end anastomosis on a rat carotid artery, eight sutures are usually enough, but additional stitches should be applied if needed. Do not hesitate to check the lumen from inside, as it is better to know whether the back wall is captured before all sutures are tightened. Usually in small vessels, walls are semitransparent, so if the needle can be seen through the wall, it means the needle is usually under only one layer, but if it is not seen, it is usually under two layers, meaning that the opposite wall of the vessel has been inadvertently captured by the needle and trapped into the knot, which should be avoided. When the anastomosis is finished, check for bleeding, achieve hemostasis as necessary, and check the blood flow through anastomosis.

You can perform multiple end-to-end anastomoses on different vessels from the same animal and combine these anastomoses with other types of anastomoses. We advise trying three different techniques for placing the stay sutures and different vessel orientations to bring variety and interest to your training sessions.

Sidebar

The vessel wall must be held *only* by the adventitia or by using the counter-press method. When the vessel wall is squeezed by the forceps, the endothelium can be damaged, leading to thrombosis.

5.3 Exercise: End-to-Side Anastomosis on Rat Carotid Arteries—Continuous Suture

This exercise simulates the technique needed to create a superficial temporal artery-to-middle cerebral artery anastomosis in the end-to-side fashion. The carotid arteries are preferred over the femoral arteries for this simulation because femoral vessels are considerably smaller than the middle cerebral arteries. This exercise can be completed twice on one animal. Because rats usually have a well-developed circle of Willis, they can easily tolerate occlusion in one carotid artery, when a survival experiment is planned.

The approach to the carotid arteries is described in Chapter 4. After the arteries are dissected free from the periadventitial tissues, one artery is chosen as a donor and another as a recipient (▶ Fig. 5.3). A stepwise description of the end-to-side anastomosis technique on rat carotid arteries is presented in ▶ Fig. 5.4. The donor artery is clipped proximally and distally, then cut at the distal end and rotated across the midline to the contralateral side. The path depends on the available length of the transferring carotid artery. A long artery can be moved across the midline in front of the trachea, while a shorter vascular pedicle can be passed behind the trachea. The distal end of the donor artery is ligated.

Linear arteriotomy on the recipient vessel is begun using an unused 27-gauge needle and continued with microscissors. The techniques for tailoring the donor vessel optimally and end-to-side anastomosis are described in Chapter 3 (▶ Fig. 3.31, ▶ Fig. 3.32). Trainees can practice classic fish-mouth tailoring first to understand how much of a toe is required to achieve an optimal angle for enlargement of the anastomosis. Heparinized

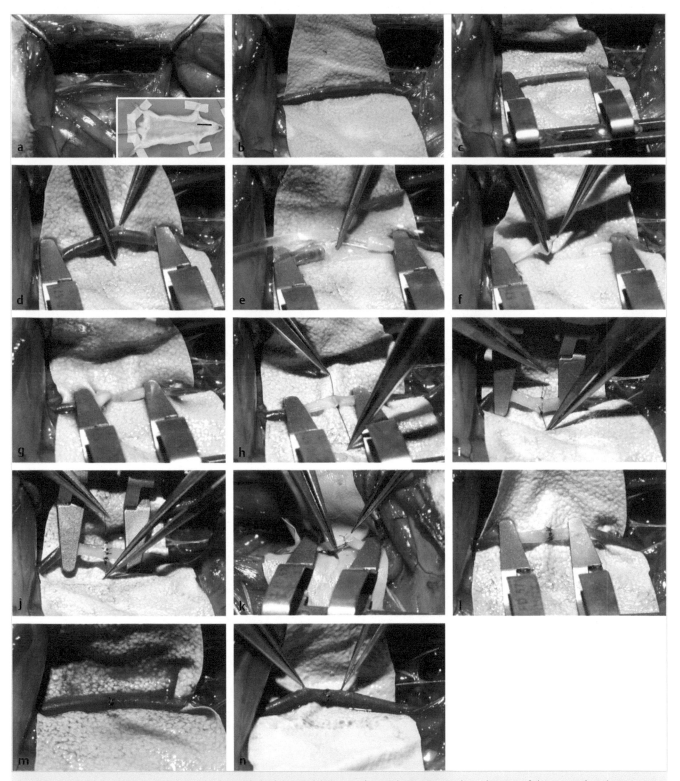

Fig. 5.2 End-to-end anastomosis on rat carotid arteries (Video 5.1). **(a)** Dissected carotid artery. Inset shows location of the approach and orientation of the operative field. **(b)** A latex background is placed under the artery. **(c)** A clip approximator is applied. **(d)** The vessel is cut at the middle and **(e)** is washed with heparinized saline. **(f)** The adventitia is gently removed from the ends of the joining vessels. **(g)** The cleaned ends are then moved closer to each other by moving one clip of the approximator. **(h)** The first two sutures are placed opposite to each other. **(i)** The clip approximator is rotated 180 degrees to show the other side of the vessels. **(j)** The back wall is sutured with separate sutures first. **(k)** The vessel lumen is checked from inside for any mistakes. **(l)** Sutures are placed on the front wall of anastomosis. **(m)** The clips are removed, and a small amount of bleeding is usually observed. **(n)** Bleeding from the needle puncture sites usually stops by itself with gentle pressure within a few minutes.

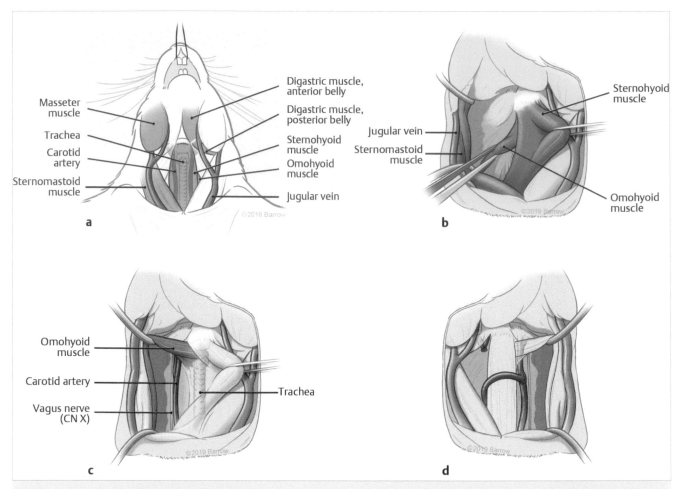

Fig. 5.3 Training on the neck vessels of a rat. **(a)** Location of the carotid artery and jugular vein in the neck. **(b)** The sternohyoid muscle is retracted medially and the sternomastoid muscle laterally. The omohyoid muscle crosses the surgical field. **(c)** The omohyoid muscle is retracted superolaterally to expose the carotid artery and vagus nerve. **(d)** End-to-side anastomosis of the distal end of the right carotid artery to the left carotid artery is shown. The proximal end of the carotid artery may also be used instead of the distal for this exercise.

saline should be used to keep the tissues moist. ▶ Fig. 5.4 and Video 5.2 show the creation of an anastomosis with continuous suture. After placing the toe and heel stay sutures, suture the back wall first and proceed with the easier front wall last. Before tying the last knot, temporarily release the distal clip to wash out possible thrombus and air.

5.4 Exercise: Double End-to-Side Anastomosis on Carotid Arteries— Arterial Loop

In this training exercise, you will create an arterial loop by performing a double end-to-side anastomosis on the carotid arteries. After completing a single end-to-side anastomosis between the left and right carotid arteries, ligate and cut the same carotid artery again, but now at its caudal end. This free end of the artery is then anastomosed to the recipient carotid artery on the opposite side, distally or proximally to the first anastomosis. After the second end-to-side anastomosis is completed, a pulsatile arterial loop is formed (▶ Fig. 5.5).

5.5 Exercise: End-to-Side Anastomosis Between Carotid Artery and Jugular Vein— Interrupted Suture

This procedure is a more complex variant of an end-to-side anastomosis, mainly because it involves the dissection and handling of veins, which are more fragile than arteries. The jugular veins lie more superficially than the carotid arteries and require

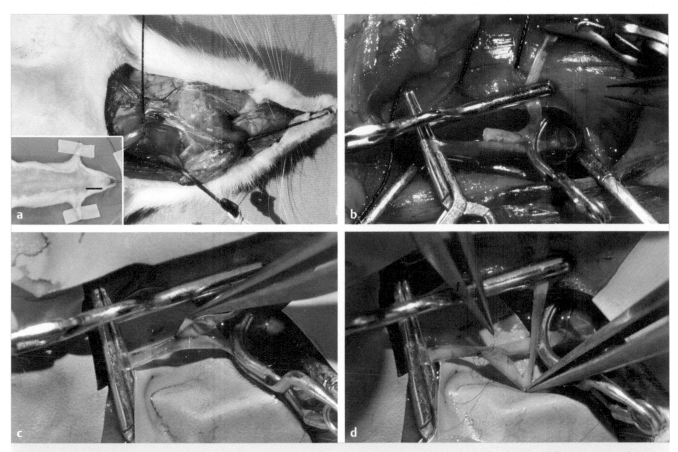

Fig. 5.4 End-to-side anastomosis on rat carotid arteries (Video 5.2). **(a)** View of animal positioning and approach to carotid arteries. Inset shows location of the approach and orientation of the operative field. **(b)** The carotid arteries are dissected on both sides; the right carotid artery is ligated proximally, translocated over the muscles on the left side, and aligned with the contralateral carotid artery. **(c)** After finishing the continuous suturing on the back wall, the lumen is checked from the inside. **(d)** The continuous sutures are tightened and secured. (*Continued*)

meticulous dissection and ligation of side branches. A stepwise description of this technique is presented in ▶ Fig. 5.6 and Video 5.3. The key points are the same as for any end-to-side anastomosis; however, in this anastomosis, it is usually difficult to estimate the final size of the vein because arterial flow will distend it, which makes it harder to prepare the appropriate side opening on the carotid artery. After the toe and heel sutures are placed, the front and back sides of the anastomosis are sutured. As can be seen in ▶ Fig. 5.6m, we used interrupted sutures. Each suture was placed and tied individually, except for the last two, which were placed without tightening, so there was enough space to place the instruments for the counterpressure technique for the last suture. Once the last suture had been placed, the knots were made.

The adventitia of veins is very thin and attaches to the fine media and intima without a clear border, so it cannot be removed as efficiently as it can from arteries. Because of this quality, removing adventitia from a vein requires more precise microdissection.

Continuous suture with loose loops makes suturing easier at the final steps. This method is especially helpful when suturing veins with their thin walls. The running suture suspends the vessel open, preventing the collapse of walls and enlarging the opening between the two vessels. The infusion of isotonic saline

can also help to prevent the vein wall from collapsing. To save time, experienced surgeons sometimes make the running suture by piercing both vessel walls with one movement of the needle. During suturing of the vessel wall, the filament should be seen through the vessel wall, which indicates the adequate coaptation of vessels with no folding of the intima.

The sutures are cut after the knots are tied, leaving 0.2-mm to 0.3-mm ends. One end can be made longer than the other, so it will be easier to grasp it with forceps when needed.

5.6 Exercise: Side-to-Side Anastomosis on a Femoral Artery and Vein—Continuous Suture

The basic technique of side-to-side anastomosis is described in Chapter 3, Section 3.8.5 Side-to-Side Anastomosis. Training of a side-to-side anastomosis requires two parallel vessels. In a biological model, you can use a naturally encountered parallel artery and vein or you can dissect an arterial graft separately on the contralateral side. For the example of this exercise, we performed side-to-side anastomosis on a rat femoral artery and vein (▶ Fig. 5.7, Video 5.4). Because of the small vessel size, we did not place a second stay suture for this anastomosis.

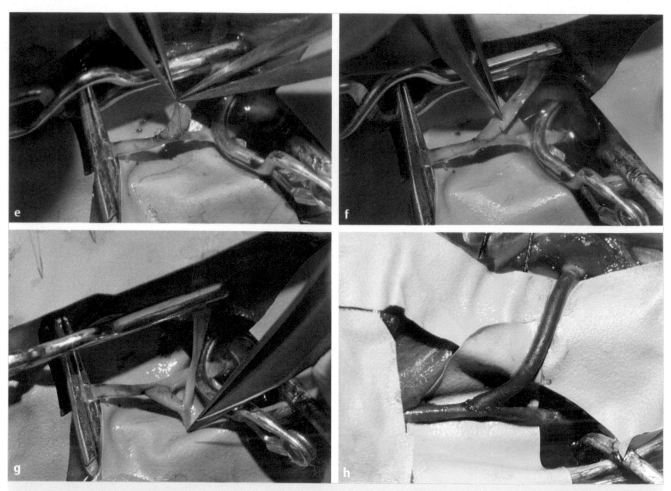

Fig. 5.4 (*Continued*) (**e**) Continuous sutures are placed on the front wall in a right-to-left direction. (**f**) The front wall sutures are tightened. (**g**) The back and front wall sutures are tightened. (**h**) View after removing the temporary clips and achieving hemostasis.

5.7 Tests for Patency of the Anastomosis

After completion, the anastomosis should be assessed visually under medium magnification of the microscope. There are several simple tests to assess patency of anastomosis. The first method is purely observational and relies on determination of one of the three types of pulsation.[5] If the anastomosis is patent, the distal artery should pulsate and slightly enlarge with every systole, that is, expansile pulsation, or it should have a "wriggling" pulsation. Pulsatile movement of the anastomosis toward the direction of flow with elongation of artery, "longitudinal pulsation" usually means that the blood flow is obstructed. Pulsation of the vessel proximal to anastomosis should never be used as a sign of patency.[5]

The "lift test" is more sensitive. The vessel is lifted from underneath with closed forceps until the blood flow stops. The artery above the forceps becomes pale. Then the forceps are moved distally to the anastomosis with the same lifting force. If the anastomosis is patent, the vessel should rapidly become filled with blood.[6]

The "milking" test (also known as Acland's test or the double occlusion test) requires two forceps. Gently squeeze the artery

distal to the anastomosis with two forceps placed close to each other. While the forceps are closed, spread them to the sides ("milking" movement), creating a bloodless segment of the artery. Then release the proximal forceps: if the arterial segment swiftly fills with the blood, then the anastomosis is patent; if it does not, there is a proximal obstruction.[5]

Squeezing the artery with the forceps may be traumatic, so the same milking test can instead be reproduced using a single angulated-tip forceps. The closed forceps are introduced underneath the vessel and used to lift the vessel until the blood flow stops. Then the forceps are opened, creating a bloodless arterial segment between the tips. Then the forceps are rotated to the side, releasing the pressure to the vessel from the proximal forceps' tip. If the vessel segment is filled with the blood, the anastomosis is patent.

Additionally, when the vessel is lifted by the forceps, one can observe the pulsation of the arterial blood, which breaks through the compressing lifting pressure of the forceps with each systole. This test relies on the flickering of arterial blood and works only on the thin-walled translucent vessels.

Finally, the patency of the anastomosis can be confirmed by ultrasound or by injecting dyes while watching for a change in color distal to the anastomosis. Nonfluorescent dyes (e.g., methylene blue) as well as fluorescent dyes (e.g., fluorescein sodium

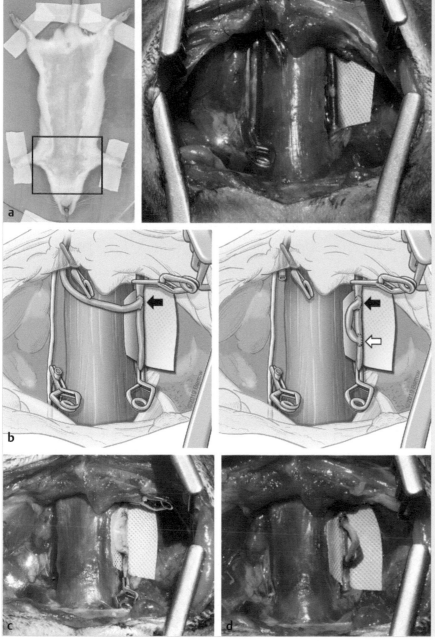

Fig. 5.5 Double end-to-side anastomosis on carotid arteries of a rat (arterial loop). **(a)** Photograph showing location of the approach and orientation of the operative field (*left*) and intraoperative photograph (*right*) of surgical exposure: the left carotid artery is prepared for harvesting, and the right carotid artery is exposed on a background. **(b)** Illustrations showing the first anastomosis created between distal end of the left carotid artery and proximal right carotid (*left, black arrow*) and the second anastomosis between proximal end of the left carotid and distal portion of the right carotid (*right, white arrow*). **(c)** Final result after completion of suturing of both anastomoses and formation of vascular loop. **(d)** Blood flow through the vessels shows the patency of both anastomoses.

and indocyanine green) can be used with the appropriate light filters on the microscope. Radiographic angiography is unnecessary in training settings; however, it can be used in chronic experiments to assess long-term patency of the anastomosis.

5.8 Hemostasis

Hemostasis can be difficult to achieve, and the anastomosis may seem leaky at first. Slight bleeding from the needle puncture sites is unavoidable and stops with time on its own. However, bleeding will persist in some cases, especially with generous use of heparin wash. Points of copious stream-like bleeding most often occur in places of unequal coaptation of the vessel edges and triangular tissue protrusions (so-called

dog ears). Very few sutures are actually needed to join the vessels without significant bleeding because blood pressure pushes the walls outward, which closes the gaps between the sutures in the same way as leaflets of the heart valves obstruct the backflow.

When bleeding occurs right after the clips are opened, the clips can be closed for a while and then opened again. While the clips are closed, one can finish tightening the final knot. This method allows the blood flow to stagnate and small clots to appear that close the small holes from the needle punctures. If oozing continues after removing the clip, apply gentle pressure with a cotton pad and wait several minutes for clot formation. If bleeding still continues, use a small piece of smashed muscle or fat to wrap around the anastomosis (► Fig. 5.8).

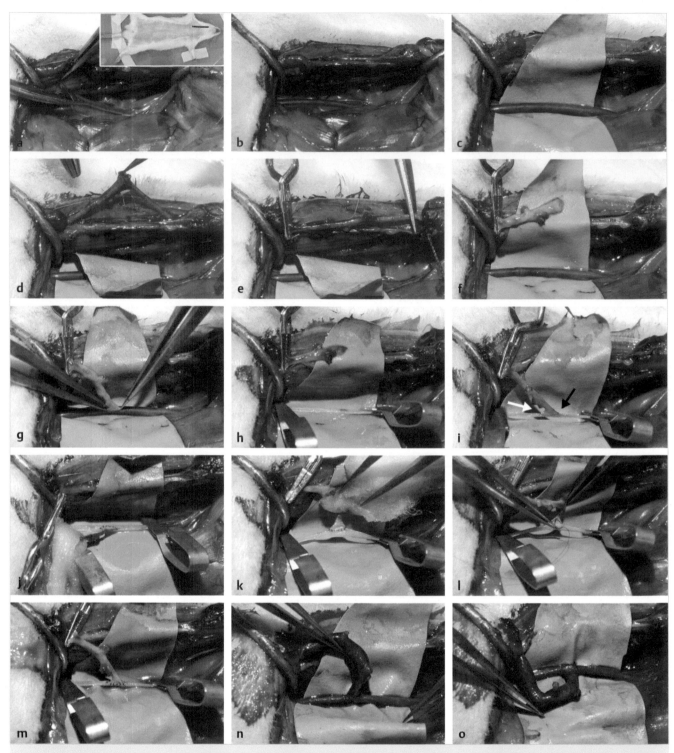

Fig. 5.6 Carotid–jugular fistula: Technique of end-to-side anastomosis of carotid and jugular vessels with interrupted suture (Video 5.3). **(a)** The carotid artery is dissected from its connective tissue. Inset shows the location of the approach and orientation of the operative field. **(b)** The right carotid artery is exposed. **(c)** A latex background is placed behind the exposed artery. **(d)** The jugular vein is carefully dissected out, coagulating side branches. **(e)** The jugular vein is coagulated and cut distally and **(f)** is washed with a heparinized solution. **(g)** The vessels are aligned to mark the sites of the planned anastomosis. **(h)** The adventitia is removed from the joining vessels, the vein is trimmed in a fish-mouth fashion, and the carotid artery is incised. **(i)** The vein is fixed with two stay sutures on toe and heel. **(j)** One side of the anastomosis is completed with interrupted sutures. **(k)** The back side of the sutured wall is checked from inside the vessel. **(l)** Image showing puncturing of both vessel walls with a single needle pass. **(m)** The front wall is finished with interrupted sutures. **(n)** Blood flow is restored when clips are removed. **(o)** The vein has become distended and bright red, showing patency of the anastomosis.

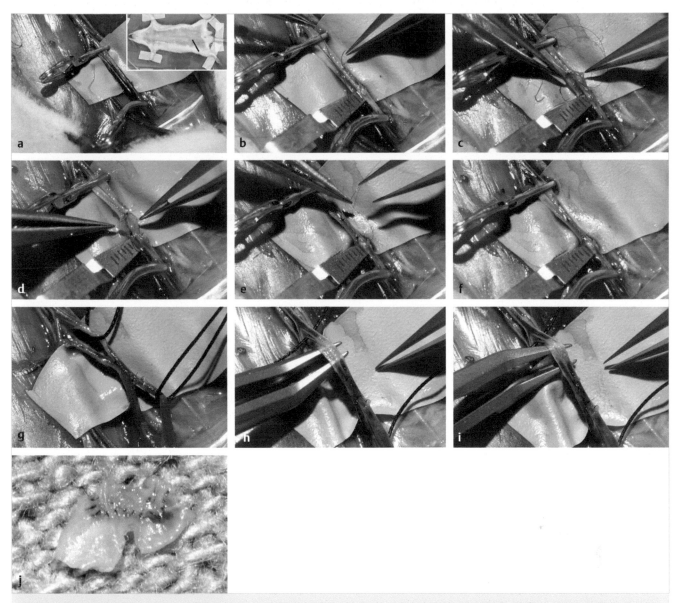

Fig. 5.7 Side-to-side anastomosis on rat femoral vessels (Video 5.4). **(a)** The femoral artery and vein are dissected and clipped in parallel to each other. A planned incision approximately 2 to 2.5 times the diameter of the vessel is marked. Inset shows location of the approach and orientation of the operative field. **(b)** The vessels are opened with 27-gauge needle and microscissors, and the first suture is applied. No second stay suture is placed on the other end because of the small vessel size. **(c)** Continuous sutures are placed on the back wall of the anastomosis from inside the lumen. **(d)** Continuous sutures are placed on the front wall of the anastomosis. **(e)** The front wall is closed with the continuous sutures in the same direction from upper left to lower right. **(f)** The suture ends are connected, tightened, and cut. **(g)** After the clips are removed, blood flow is restored, and arterialization of the vein is observed. **(h)** By gently compressing the vessels with a lifting movement of forceps and moving the forceps (lift test), **(i)** the blood flow filling the vessel is observed, confirming patency of the anastomosis. **(j)** The resected anastomosis site is checked under the microscope for any mistakes.

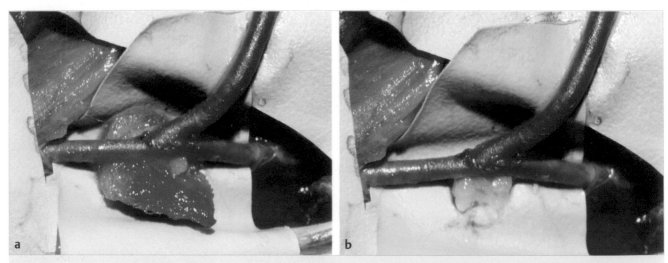

Fig. 5.8 Hemostasis may be successfully facilitated with **(a)** a cottonoid or **(b)** placement of fat or crushed muscle tissue on the bleeding spots.

Crushed tissue provides plenty of coagulation factors and facilitates clot formation. If none of these measures work, or if the bleeding is brisk, additional sutures should be placed.

References

[1] Belykh E, Lei T, Safavi-Abbasi S, et al. Low-flow and high-flow neurosurgical bypass and anastomosis training models using human and bovine placental vessels: a histological analysis and validation study. J Neurosurg; 125(4):915–928

[2] Chase MD, Schwartz SI, Rob C. A technique of small artery anastomosis. Surg Gynecol Obstet; 116:381–384

[3] Cobbett J. Small vessel anastomosis. A comparison of suture techniques. Br J Plast Surg; 20(1):16–20

[4] Fujino T, Aoyagi F. A method of successive interrupted suturing in microvascular anastomoses. Plast Reconstr Surg; 55(2):240–241

[5] Acland R. Signs of patency in small vessel anastomosis. Surgery; 72(5):744–748

[6] MacDonald JD. Learning to perform microvascular anastomosis. Skull Base; 15(3):229–240

6 Day 5: Exercise Set 2: Deep Field Anastomoses and Complex Vascular Reconstructions

Evgenii Belykh and Nicolay L. Martirosyan

Abstract

This chapter describes microneurosurgical exercises with an advanced level of complexity. These exercises include sharp microdissection of biological microarteries with a suction device and bayonetted microsurgical scissors, anastomoses performed in the deep operative field, several complex vascular reconstructions, and nerve suturing.

Keywords: deep surgical field, fistula, anastomosis, microdissection, sharp dissection, vascular reconstruction

6.1 Microsurgical Training in a Deep Surgical Field

Each of the techniques described in this chapter should be mastered using both short and long microsurgery instruments. A deep surgical corridor can be simulated using different tools. The basic exercises to be practiced in deep field include dissection, tying knots on gauze, and performing anastomoses (both wet and dry laboratory training). For example, an end-to-side anastomosis can be performed on silicone tubes that are placed in a model of a skull (about 6 cm deep). A skull model with a craniotomy limits the possible movements of the instruments and the hands (▶ Fig. 6.1). We have found plastic toy building bricks (Lego, The Lego Group) to be very convenient for assembling customized stands that can be used to help simulate the restrictions of working through a craniotomy and at depth in the surgical field during these exercises (▶ Fig. 6.2).

6.2 Exercise: Deep Operative Field Dissection

The deep operative field dissection exercise is essential for microneurosurgical training. It must be mastered because the skills of sharp dissection in a deep operative wound are among the most essential for successful performance of microneurosurgical procedures in patients.

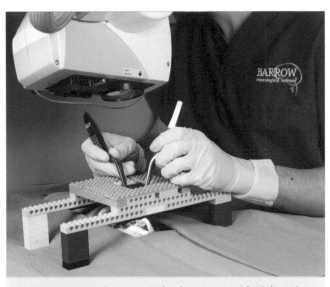

Fig. 6.2 Microsurgical practice in the deep operative field through a small opening in a stand made of plastic toy building bricks.

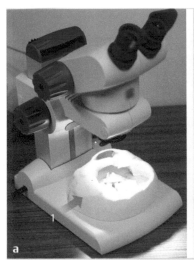
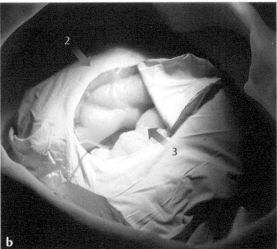
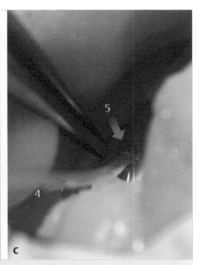

Fig. 6.1 Simulation of deep surgical wound conditions. **(a)** A model of the skull with a craniotomy (1) is placed under the stereomicroscope. **(b)** A surgical glove (2) is pulled over a silicone model of the brain (3) to simulate the dura. It is opened in a horseshoe fashion (exercise 1). **(c)** A donor artery (4) is used to perform an anastomosis with a recipient artery (5) (using 1-mm-diameter silicone tubes) deep in the cerebral sulcus. (Images provided courtesy of Evgenii Belykh, MD.)

The following materials are necessary to perform the deep operative field dissection exercise:

1. A customized stand, up to 10 cm in height, with an opening about 4 cm above the planned abdominal approach. The depth between the laboratory animal and the opening in the stand should be about 6 cm, which corresponds to the depth of the center of the skull base.
2. Bayonetted microsurgery instruments of the appropriate length: needle holder, forceps, and scissors
3. A microscope objective lens with a focal length of not less than 270 mm. Note that small laboratory stereomicroscopes may not have enough focal distance to allow dissection in a simulated deep operative field.
4. Laboratory animal (e.g., rat) or other simulation model

After the rat is anesthetized, a median laparotomy is performed. The contents of the abdominal cavity are then carefully removed, retracted to the left, and placed on the moistened gauze.

Use bayonetted microsurgery scissors to perform sharp dissection and a suction tip to apply counterpressure. Then separate the abdominal aorta from the neighboring vena cava (▶ Fig. 6.3, Video 6.1).

6.3 Exercise: Anastomosis in a Deep Operative Field

Neurosurgical trainees should have technical practice in performing microvascular anastomoses in a deep operative field. There are several clinical situations in which such skills are indispensable, such as anastomoses inside the interhemispheric fissure or deep inside the sylvian fissure and subtemporal approaches or anastomoses involving posterior fossa arteries. For experimental surgery in the laboratory setting, these situations can be simulated using a special stand to support the hands and to increase the depth of the operative field (▶ Fig. 6.4).

Training for conducting anastomoses in the deep operative field can be done using any type of blood vessel. Rat carotids may be preferable to other rat vessels because their size more nearly matches the cerebral arteries of the human patient than other alternatives. However, exercises on the rat femoral vascular bundle are more demanding and therefore more challenging for training. For example, we describe an end-to-side anastomosis on a femoral vascular bundle that creates an arteriovenous fistula (▶ Fig. 6.5).

The femoral vascular bundle is dissected in a standard fashion, and a small triangle of colored latex (i.e., a piece of a surgical glove) is placed under the vessels for better visualization. The temporary clips are applied to both the artery and the vein approximately 1 cm apart from each other. The end-to-side (end of artery to side of vein) anastomosis is then created using interrupted sutures. It is easier to make the opening in the vein when a traction suture is applied first to lift the vessel wall. The vein opening should not be too long, however, because the vein tends to collapse and shrink without the tension provided by blood flow. On the bloodless vein, the length of the incision may look appropriate, but it distends with arterial pressure, which can result in a much larger opening than originally thought.

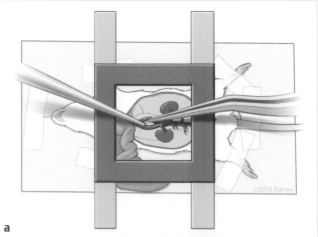

a

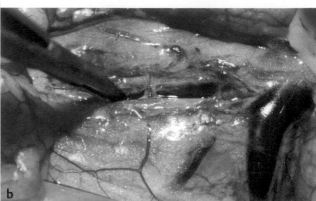

b

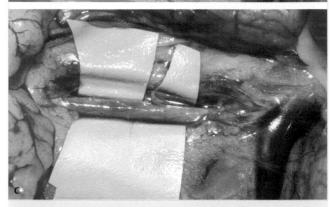

c

Fig. 6.3 Dissection of the aorta from the vena cava in a deep operative field (Video 6.1). **(a)** Illustration demonstrates the limitations of the surgical field and dissection of the vessels with a suction tip and microforceps. **(b)** Overview of the aorta and vena cava beneath the retroperitoneal fat tissue. **(c)** Dissected aorta is placed on a piece of colored latex to aid visualization.

To avoid a mismatch of the joining vessels, mark the planned arteriotomies on the distended vessels. Before tying the last suture, release the distal clip temporarily to wash out any thromboses and air. Then release the proximal clip temporarily for the same purpose before finally tying the last suture. After the anastomosis is completed, remove the distal clip first. Blood will fill the vein and the artery up to the arterial clip, which will then reveal any leakage. To stop a leak, place additional stitches at the site of the leak. In the final step, remove the arterial clip

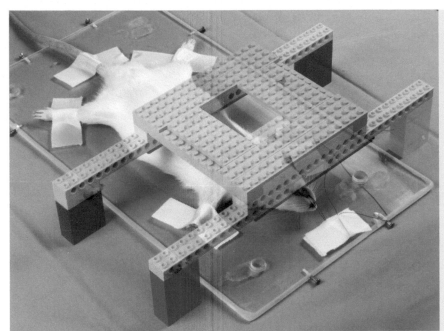

Fig. 6.4 A stand made with plastic toy building blocks with a small elevated opening can be used to simulate a deep operative field for practicing microneurosurgical exercises using anesthetized laboratory animals.

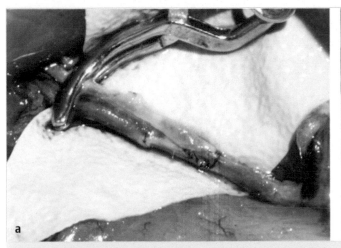
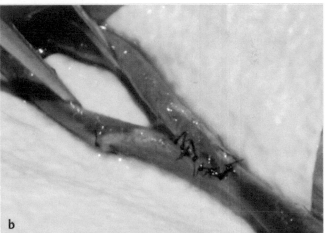

Fig. 6.5 Arteriovenous fistula created by an end-to-side anastomosis using the end of an artery and the side of a vein. **(a)** After the anastomosis is complete, a distal clip is removed from the vein. The vein is dark blue; the artery is pink. **(b)** After the proximal clip is removed from the artery, the vein fills with arterial blood, turns red, and expands in diameter.

to allow the vein to fill with arterial blood, which causes it to become red and pulsatile. The change in color and the pulsation of the vein confirm the patency of the anastomosis.

6.4 Complex Microvascular Reconstruction

Cerebrovascular neurosurgeons must be ready to apply their microsurgical suturing skills in all sorts of demanding intraoperative situations. Sometimes doing so requires creativity and nonstandard solutions (thinking outside the box). One such technically demanding solution is anastomosis between the end of an individual donor artery and the ends of two recipient arteries (▶ Fig. 6.6).[1]

There are many options for complex vascular reconstructions to suit the individual anatomy of a particular patient and clinical situation. One challenge is to try to reproduce such complex combinations of bypasses. For a general classification of bypass types, see Chapter 10, Translation of Laboratory Skills: Indications for Bypass in Neurosurgery.

6.5 Exercise: Mismatched Orifices —Venous Interposition Graft onto the Carotid Artery

The venous interposition graft is an exercise that is useful for learning how to anastomose microvessels of various diameters (i.e., mismatched orifices) (▶ Fig. 6.7, Video 6.2). This exercise is

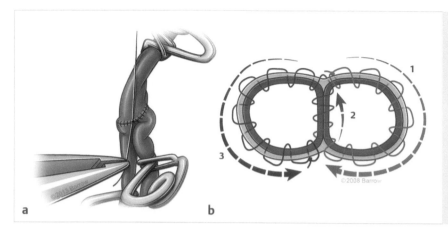

Fig. 6.6 Complex anastomosis of the end of one artery to the ends of two arteries of smaller diameter. **(a)** Illustration provides an overview of the anastomosis. **(b)** Illustration depicts directions of continuous sutures.

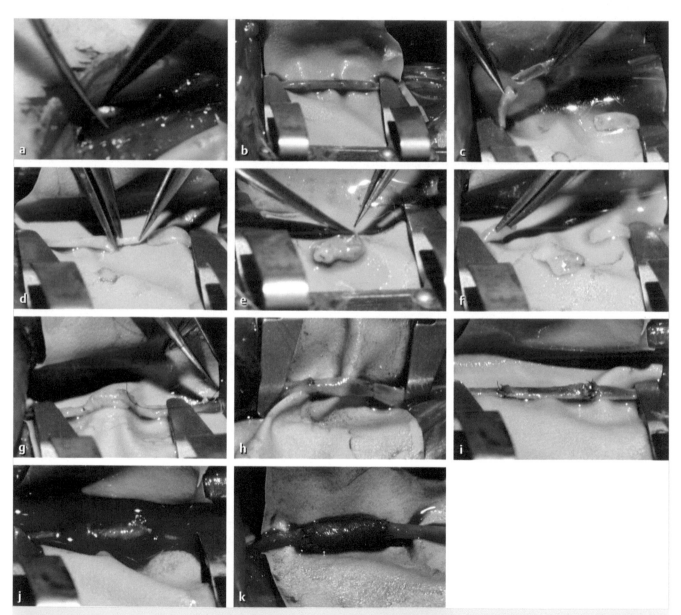

Fig. 6.7 Venous interposition graft (Video 6.2). **(a)** Segment of jugular vein is harvested. **(b)** Ipsilateral carotid artery is exposed, clipped, and cut in half. **(c)** Arterial ends are washed with heparinized solution. **(d)** Arterial ends are dissected from adventitia. **(e)** Segment of vein is washed and cleaned of adventitia. **(f)** Arterial vessels are enlarged using a fish-mouth technique. **(g)** Venous graft is first fixed with four stay sutures, one each at the four corners. **(h)** Both back walls are sutured first with interrupted sutures. **(i)** The vessel lumen is checked from inside before suturing the front wall. **(j)** Clips are removed, which results in oozing of blood. **(k)** View of vascular graft after hemostasis has been achieved.

one of the most demanding because it requires not only perfect suturing skills but also gentle handling of tissues to work with venous grafts and advanced tailoring skills to match the diameters of arterial and vein openings. Even small mistakes usually lead to graft thrombosis because of the turbulent flow in an enlarged graft. The most critical part is to mentally calculate the distended vein diameter and then trim the arterial ends accordingly. After finishing both anastomoses, you can observe pronounced pulsation of the graft. This exercise will show how a graft taken from the jugular vein might be a huge size mismatch to the carotid artery. In contrast, a segment of femoral vein with a smaller diameter can be harvested to provide a good match in size.

6.6 Exercise: Epineural Suture

Microsurgical nerve repair is performed in many surgical specialties. Although tunnel grafts are increasingly popular for nerve repair, every neurosurgeon should be ready to perform neurorrhaphy in both planned and emergency cases. Such training would likely help improve treatment outcomes in patients with peripheral nerve lesions and decrease the number of reoperations and complicated secondary reconstructions. Epineural and fascicular nerve repair skills can be obtained only in the microsurgical laboratory. The neural sheath is an extremely fragile structure, and special training is required to learn how to handle it appropriately.

Training on nerve repair is usually performed on the femoral nerve of the rat, which runs along the femoral vessels. The femoral nerve is dissected off the femoral vessels, and a piece of latex is placed beneath it for better visualization. Before cutting across the nerve, you should carefully examine the surface (i.e., the epineurium) under high magnification to help you remember the orientation of the bundles, so they can be placed in the correct position when anastomosing.

To suture the epineurium, you make the first "bite" at the edge of the nerve and immediately push the needle up to prevent damage to the fascicles (▶ Fig. 6.8). The movement of the needle resembles the motion of an airplane takeoff. You then make the next bite just beneath the epineurium. Push the needle deeper along the axis of the nerve and then out. Tie the suture loosely, just for approximation of the stumps and to prevent rotation, bending, and bulging. Make the second stitch 120 degrees from the first one. Then gently rotate the nerve to apply a third stitch.

Sidebar

- For a small (< 1 mm) nerve, three sutures should be adequate to ensure the appropriate orientation of the ends. Limiting the number of sutures also helps prevent scarring.

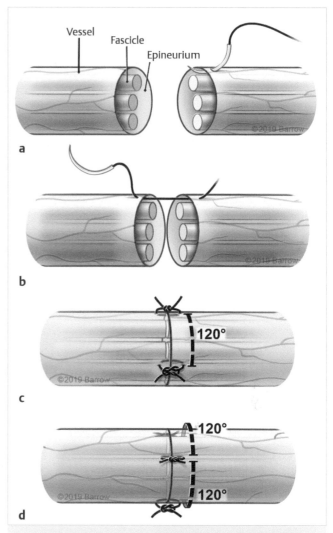

Fig. 6.8 Application of an epineural suture. Illustration depicts **(a)** first bite of the needle for the first suture; **(b)** passage of the needle through the opposite nerve end; **(c)** completion of a second stitch, which is tied loosely like the first; and **(d)** gentle rotation of the nerve to allow placement of a third stitch, if necessary. Three sutures placed evenly on the circumference are 120 degrees apart from each other.

6.7 Exercise: Fascicular Suture

Although fascicular nerve repair is performed only on rare occasions in neurosurgical practice, it is an interesting exercise (▶ Fig. 6.9). After placing the femoral nerve on the colored latex background and cutting it transversely, remove a tiny amount of epineurium from both neural ends. Corresponding fascicles should be recognizable under the highest magnification.

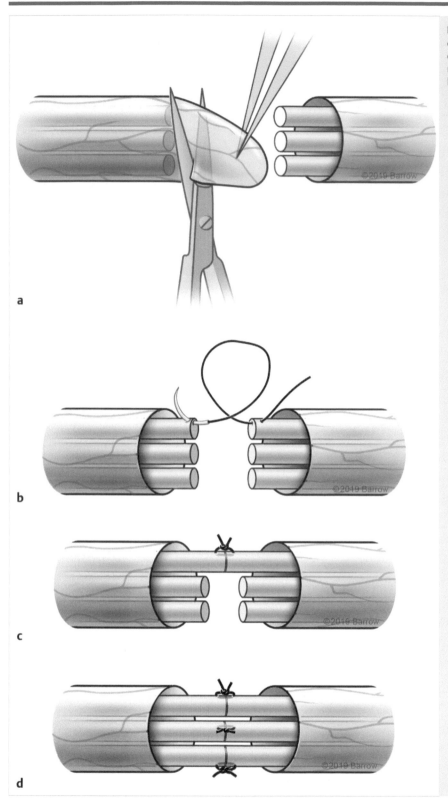

Fig. 6.9 Fascicular nerve repair. Illustration depicts **(a)** removal of a short segment of epineurium; **(b)** entering and exit bites of the needle for the first stitch; **(c)** first stitch, tied loosely; and **(d)** one stitch for each fascicle.

a

b

c

d

Use a tiny (10–0 suturing) needle to enter the fascicle at a 45-degree angle close to the edge. After the first bite, push the needle parallel to the fascicle to minimize intraneural damage. Tie the sutures loosely to prevent scarring. For fascicles that are less than 0.5 mm in diameter, one suture should be enough for each fascicle. However, an additional suture can be added, if necessary.

Reference

[1] Spetzler RF, Rhoton AL, Nakaji P, Kawashima M. Color Atlas of Cerebral Revascularization. New York, NY: Thieme Medical Publishers; 2013

7 Day 6: Exercises: Kidney Autotransplantation, Supermicrosurgery, and Aneurysm Clipping

Evgenii Belykh and Nikolay L. Martirosyan

Abstract

In the later stages of microsurgical training, when your skills are plateauing, challenging yourself with a complex microsurgical procedure can further improve your abilities. In this chapter, we present the concept of supermicrosurgery and a rat kidney autotransplantation exercise to help develop necessary tissue handling and anastomosis skills. We also provide an introduction to aneurysm clipping.

Keywords: aneurysm, autotransplantation, clipping, kidney, placenta, supermicrosurgery

7.1 Exercise: Kidney Autotransplantation

Kidney transplantation in a rat is a technically demanding exercise that microsurgeons are often required to master. This exercise consists of three anastomoses: arterial, venous, and ureteral. In this case, a kidney may be transplanted to either the femoral vascular bundle or the aorta (▶ Fig. 7.1).

Renal autotransplantation is a time-consuming staged procedure that requires good anastomosis skills, respectful tissue handling, and advanced planning (▶ Fig. 7.2). To begin the procedure, a median laparotomy is performed. The left kidney is then identified, and the ureter is found by its peristaltic movements and is dissected bluntly. The pararenal soft tissues are removed, and the renal vascular pedicle is thoroughly dissected to prepare the vessels for anastomosis. Proximal clips are applied, and the vessels are cut, leaving a stump that is long enough to allow anastomosis to be performed. The ureter should be cut near the distal end. Next, the kidney is perfused through the renal artery with ice-cold normal saline. First, the renal vein is anastomosed in the end-to-side fashion, and then the arterial anastomosis is performed using the same technique.

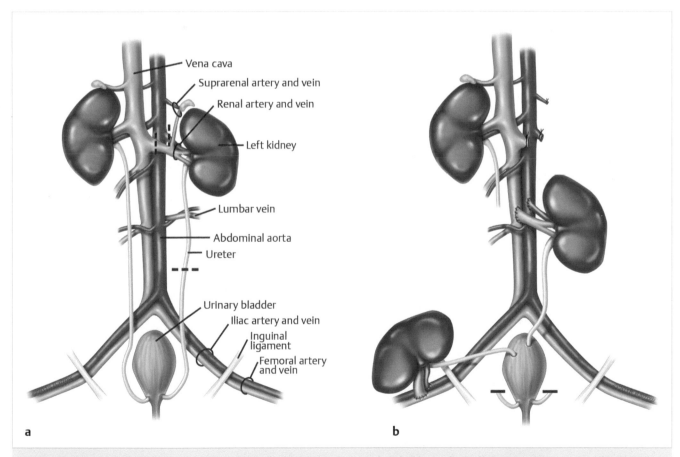

Fig. 7.1 Illustration showing kidney autotransplantation. **(a)** Left kidney is harvested; *dashed lines* indicate the location of the incisions. **(b)** Kidney may be anastomosed to the femoral vessels or aorta and vena cava. The *black bars* indicate the location of the ureter incisions.

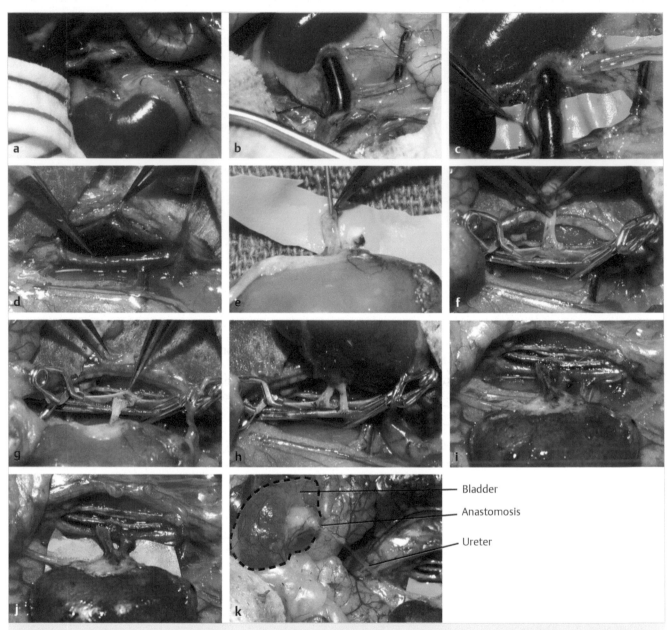

Fig. 7.2 Stepwise illustration of kidney autotransplantation. **(a)** The right kidney is exposed, revealing a short vascular pedicle. **(b)** In both rats and humans, the left kidney has a longer vascular pedicle than does the right kidney. **(c)** The left renal artery, vein, and ureter are dissected. **(d)** The aorta and vena cava segments are dissected in preparation for anastomosis. **(e)** The kidney is washed with ice-cold normal saline, the renal artery and vein are cleaned of adventitia, and the kidney parenchyma has become pale. **(f)** The aorta and vena cava are clipped, and the front wall of the venous anastomosis is finished first, leaving space for the arterial anastomosis between the clips. **(g)** The venous anastomosis is checked from the inside, and then the back wall is sutured. **(h)** The arterial anastomosis is created at a different level than the venous anastomosis for convenience. **(i)** The clips are removed, and blood flow is restored. **(j)** Note that the kidney parenchyma regains a red color after restoration of blood flow. **(k)** The ureter is inserted into the bladder through a small incision and fixed with a pair of sutures. Peristalsis should be observed (Video 7.1).

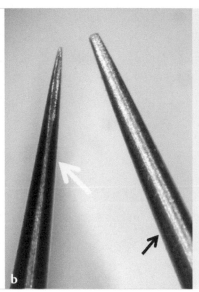

Fig. 7.3 **(a)** Sutures, needles, and **(b)** forceps used for supermicrosurgery (*yellow arrows*) and microsurgery (*black arrows*). (Reproduced with permission from Mihara et al.[2])

7.2 Exercise: Supermicrosurgery to Create a Free Groin Flap with the Vascular Pedicle

Supermicrosurgery is defined as the technique employed in the anastomosis of vessels less than 1 mm in diameter.[1] This surgical technique allows surgeons to perform vascularized flap transplantation, fingertip transplantation, lymphovenous anastomoses for edema treatment, and experimental studies on the transplantation of vascularized tissues and organs in laboratory animals. In neurosurgery, anastomoses are performed on vessels of such small diameters for the treatment of moyamoya disease in children. The performance of supermicrosurgery requires instruments with ultrasmall tips (e.g., 0.06-mm forceps tips compared with the average microsurgery forceps tips of 0.15 mm), 0.05-mm needles (12–0), and a special operative microscope with 50x magnification (▶ Fig. 7.3).[2]

Finding small vessels with a diameter of less than 1 mm for practice is easy in many animal models. One classic example used for supermicrosurgical training is the creation of an epigastric artery flap.[3] In this exercise, a rat is anesthetized and positioned for surgery. A skin flap approximately 3 × 3 cm is dissected out and elevated on the vascular pedicle containing the inferior epigastric artery (0.3–0.4 mm in diameter) and vein (0.6–0.8 mm in diameter). These vessels arise from the femoral vessels approximately 1 cm distal to the inguinal ligament. To avoid twisting of the vascular pedicle, inferior epigastric vessels should not be freely dissected from the surrounding tissues. The vascular pedicle is treated with 2% lidocaine and kept in moistened gauze for 20 minutes, which decreases vascular spasm.[1] After the flap vitality is confirmed, the vessels are cut, and the blood is carefully removed from the flap by perfusing the flap with the ice-cold heparinized normal saline. The vessel stumps are washed with a heparinized solution and prepared for end-to-end anastomosis. Ultrasmall 11–0 or 12–0 sutures are used to create the anastomosis on such small vessels, employing greater than 25x magnification. Four sutures are usually sufficient for an arterial anastomosis, whereas 6 sutures are necessary for a venous anastomosis. After the anastomosis is checked for patency, the skin flap is sutured back in place. In this survival experiment, the quality of the anastomosis is assessed daily until the wound is healed or the flap is rejected.

7.3 Exercise: Aneurysm Dissection and Clipping in a Human Placenta Model

Aneurysm clipping is a challenging surgical procedure for treating ruptured or unruptured aneurysms. A human placenta attached to a colored pressurized flow device is a good model for training in microdissection and clip application to learn to apply differently shaped clips in various positions.[4] Additionally, aneurysms can be surgically created in vivo or ex vivo in any other vessels by suturing venous or arterial patches to the arterial wall. In the placenta model, narrow- and wide-neck aneurysms can be created in the surface arteries with an intravascular balloon and branch ligation (▶ Fig. 7.4).[4] Sharp aneurysm dissection and application of various types of clips may be practiced on this model. Clip application techniques have been described in great detail by Lawton.[5] Simple clipping (▶ Fig. 7.5) with a single clip is a straightforward technique when the clip is placed across the neck of an aneurysm. One should pay close attention to even closure of the clips at their distal tip, completeness of neck closure, and the absence of "dog-ear" remnants, which may become a nidus for aneurysm regrowth.

Some aneurysms require clipping with multiple clipping strategies (▶ Fig. 7.6, ▶ Fig. 7.7), such as the use of intersecting clips, parallel clips, tandem clips, fenestrated clips to create a tube, tandem clipping with fenestrated angled clips, and clipping with wrapping.[5] *Angled fenestrated clips* can be placed in a single or tandem fashion to close challenging aneurysm domes projecting behind the parent vessel (▶ Fig. 7.6a, ▶ Fig. 7.7a). The *intersecting* clipping technique is a two-clip technique in which an intersection is created when a subsequent clip is placed at

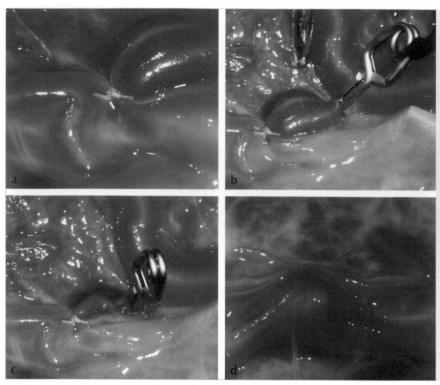

Fig. 7.4 Training for aneurysm clipping using a human placenta. **(a)** An aneurysm is created by intravascular inflation of a balloon from a small urinary catheter. After the vessel wall is remodeled, a side branch is ligated to produce an aneurysm-like structure. **(b)** Clip application. **(c)** The aneurysm is deflated by puncturing it to show complete clipping without residual flow. **(d)** Fusiform aneurysm model created by intravascular balloon inflation.

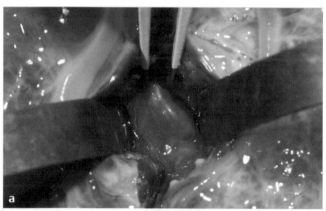

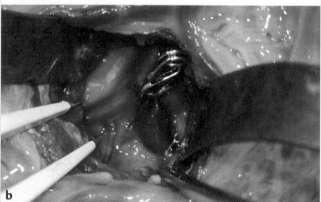

Fig. 7.5 Simple clipping of an aneurysm in a placenta model. **(a)** Preparation for clipping. **(b)** After clip placement.

an angle to the preceding adjacent clip and touches it to close off an aneurysm (▶ Fig. 7.6b, ▶ Fig. 7.7b). The *parallel* clipping (palisading stacked clips) technique may be performed in two ways: (1) *overstacking*, in which the first clip occludes most of the neck and the subsequent clips are stacked in parallel toward the aneurysm body to occlude the remaining neck, and (2) *understacking*, in which the first clip is applied to the neck on the aneurysm body and each subsequent clip is stacked toward the vessel, which produces progressively contoured aneurysm closure while the preceding clips prevent slippage. For the *overlapping* clipping method, a fenestrated clip is applied for the closure of a deep aneurysmal remnant, and the tips of the previous clip remain within the fenestration (▶ Fig. 7.6c, ▶ Fig. 7.7c). For *tandem* clipping, a straight fenestrated clip is applied to close the deep part of the aneurysm first, and simple clips are then used to close the remaining part of the aneurysm within the fenestration window.[5] An arterial branch can be preserved using clip *fenestration*. Subsequent clips can be applied in an understacked (▶ Fig. 7.6d, ▶ Fig. 7.7d) or overstacked (▶ Fig. 7.6e, ▶ Fig. 7.7e) fashion. Additionally, *aneurysm wrapping* with a Gore-Tex (Gore Medical) reinforcement sleeve may be practiced (▶ Fig. 7.6f, ▶ Fig. 7.7f).

To further increase the complexity of the exercises and their similarity to actual surgical conditions, two placentas can be mounted on one another to simulate the sylvian fissure dissection on the overlying placenta while clipping the aneurysm created on the surface of the underlying placenta. Additionally, a restriction device, similar to the one used to produce deep-field simulation, can be placed over the placenta for simulation of a craniotomy (▶ Fig. 7.5). Aneurysm rupture can also be simu-

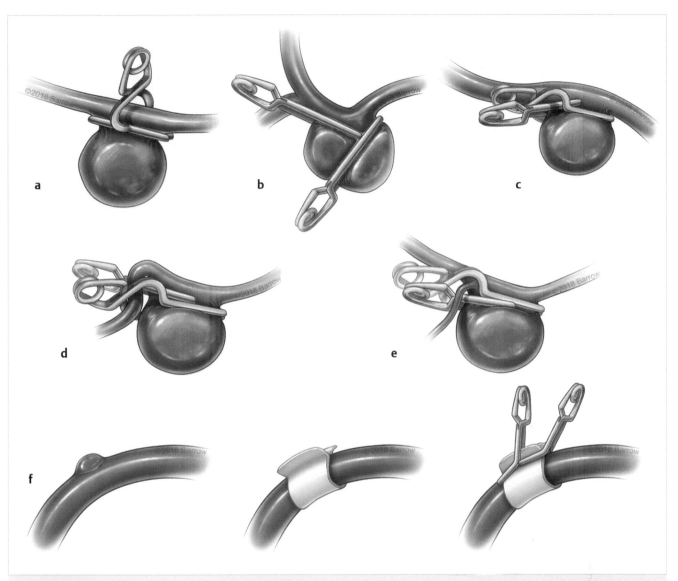

Fig. 7.6 Illustrations depicting multiple clipping techniques. **(a)** Angled fenestrated clipping. **(b)** Intersecting clipping. **(c)** An overlapping fenestrated clip is placed over a straight clip. **(d)** Tandem clipping with use of the understacking technique. **(e)** Tandem clipping with a fenestrated clip placed to save an arterial branch in the fenestration window. **(f)** Wrapping of an artery bearing a small blister-type aneurysm.

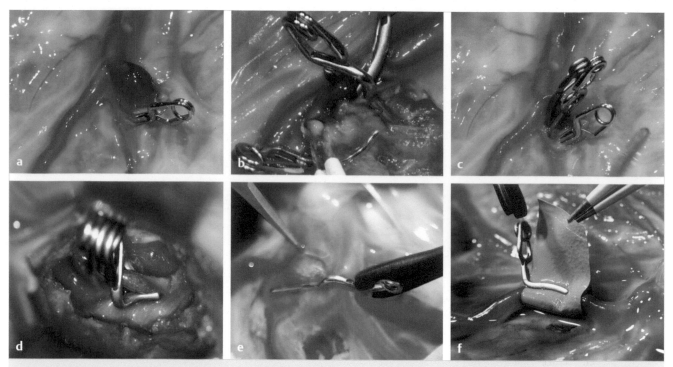

Fig. 7.7 Photographs depicting multiple clipping techniques demonstrated with use of a human placenta model. **(a)** Aneurysm is dissected, and a small bleeding point is occluded with a curved clip. **(b)** An overlapping fenestrated clip is placed over a curved clip. **(c)** Intersecting clipping. **(d)** Tandem clipping with use of the understacking technique. **(e)** Fenestrated clip placed to save an arterial branch in the fenestration window. **(f)** Wrapping of an artery bearing a small blister-type aneurysm.

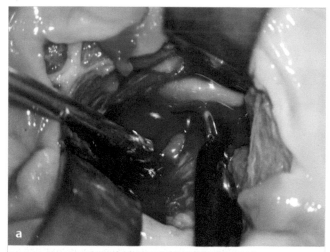

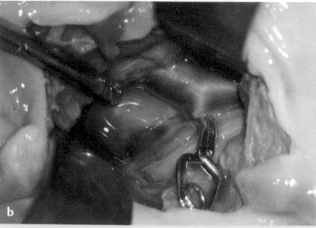

Fig. 7.8 Clipping of a ruptured aneurysm in a placental model. **(a)** Copious bleeding is controlled by suction. **(b)** The aneurysm is clipped and collapsed.

lated, which provides an opportunity to practice techniques for intraoperative bleeding control (▶ Fig. 7.8).[4]

References

[1] Mofikoya BO, Ugburo AO, Bankole OB. Microvascular anastomosis of vessels less than 0.5 mm in diameter: a supermicrosurgery training model in Lagos, Nigeria. J Hand Microsurg; 3(1):15–17

[2] Mihara M, Hayashi Y, Iida T, Narushima M, Koshima I. Instruments for supermicrosurgery in Japan. Plast Reconstr Surg; 129(2):404e–406e

[3] Ruby LK, Greene M, Risitano G, Torrejon R, Belsky MR. Experience with epigastric free flap transfer in the rat: technique and results. Microsurgery; 5(2): 102–104

[4] Oliveira Magaldi M, Nicolato A, Godinho JV, et al. Human placenta aneurysm model for training neurosurgeons in vascular microsurgery. Neurosurgery; 10 Suppl 4:592–600, discussion 600–601

[5] Lawton MT. Seven Aneurysms: Tenets and Techniques for Clipping. New York, NY: Thieme; 2010

8 Day 7: Models for Microneurosurgical Training and Schedules for Training

Evgenii Belykh, Vadim A. Byvaltsev, Mark C. Preul, and Peter Nakaji

Abstract

This chapter covers various convenient and readily available models for microneurosurgical training. We also discuss training schedules and approaches to help trainees maintain a regular schedule for training.

Keywords: bypass, chicken, model, placenta, silicone, training

8.1 Models for Microneurosurgical Training

Each bypass technique and exercise described in previous chapters can be performed on various microsurgical training models. Several models have been described in the literature, so trainees or laboratories will be able to find suitable models that meet local circumstances, budgets, and cultural and logistical requirements. In addition to models for bypass training, there are models that allow the practice of relevant neurosurgical, microsurgical, and general surgical skills.

Training can be performed as either dry-laboratory training or wet-laboratory training. *Dry-laboratory training* uses inanimate models, and *wet-laboratory training* uses live laboratory animals or human biological material. We believe that there is no single best model for bypass surgery training, as each model has its pros and cons, but it is important for a neurosurgical trainee to be aware of the alternatives and to use what is practically available.

8.1.1 Dry-Laboratory Training

Many training centers use silicone tubing to model blood vessels to help students perfect their suturing techniques at the beginning of microsurgical training. Synthetic models are recommended for studying the basic steps and techniques of performing different types of anastomoses. Dry training may be included in the curriculum for beginning students and for the first day of intensive microsurgical courses.

The primary disadvantage of synthetic models is that they do not allow the student to feel the real resistance and tension that living tissue provides when the student is practicing suturing, dissecting, and tightening knots. For this reason, nonliving tissue models can be used in the later stages of dry training after the theoretical basics and sequence of surgical steps has been covered.

Laboratory animals should not be used in the first few days of training for several reasons. First, at the beginning of training, working under "real" conditions is not so important; second, ethical guidelines favor reducing the use of animals; and third, using fewer animals will reduce the cost of training. Dry training may also be useful in the later stages of training when the same anastomosis is to be performed in a deep operative field

or other inconvenient environment where the instrument positions and moves differ from what was initially mastered.

After trainees study the technique of performing microanastomosis on nonliving tissue models, they can begin to practice on live animals. It is better to use recycled laboratory animal material from the training of more experienced trainees first, as prepared animals can be kept refrigerated (at about 4 °C) for up to 1 week after defrosting without losing the natural elasticity of the tissues.

Pressurized Models

Any dissected vessel from a chicken, turkey, placenta, or cadaver can be connected to a pressurized flow device to simulate blood flow. The easiest and least expensive solution is to use an intravenous cannula with a large syringe. Constant prolonged flow may be simulated using a pressure bag and tubing for intra-arterial infusions. Another method is to use a mechanical infusion pump that can provide arterial-like pulsatile flow.

Blood-Like Solutions

When working with nonliving models, pressurized flow aims to provide tactile feedback when working with vessels to show inadvertent vessel injury with simulated bleeding. Pressurized flow also serves as a model to practice mechanical hemostasis and to show bypass patency and major leaks near the anastomosis. Blood-like solutions for simulation should ideally be nontransparent, red, and inexpensive. We find that gouache paint diluted with water makes a good nontoxic, opaque blood-like solution.

Poultry Arteries

Chicken wings and legs are easily accessible material for learning to perform microvascular anastomoses[1,2] (▶ Fig. 8.1). A characteristic of tissue that is not fixed in formalin is that it dries out quickly; therefore, the anastomosed vessels should be regularly moistened with an isotonic solution. Turkey wings and necks have larger arteries than chicken wings and necks. The turkey arteries are similar in diameter to the human middle cerebral artery and superficial temporal artery and may also be used for microsurgical practice.[3,4]

8.1.2 Wet Training

For optimal use of laboratory animals, a single animal may be used to perform several different anastomoses. Bypass exercises can also be performed on tissue-based models other than live laboratory animals.

Cadaveric Vessels

Laboratories with access to cadavers can use cadaveric vessels of different origins, including the mesentery, peripheral

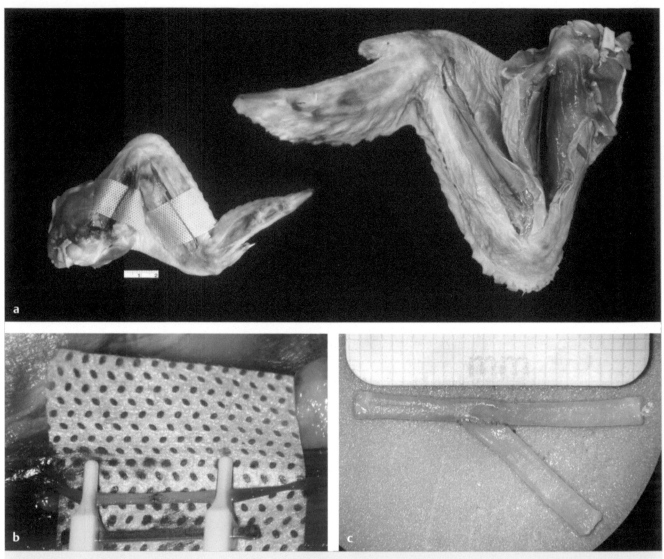

Fig. 8.1 Microsurgical training in a poultry model. **(a)** Comparison of chicken and turkey wings and usable lengths of arteries. **(b)** End-to-end anastomosis of chicken arteries. **(c)** End-to-side anastomosis of turkey arteries.

circulation, and brain,[5] to teach students the skills of microvascular anastomosis. Any human autopsy or biopsy surgical material should be used with the appropriate approval of the institution's ethics committee. Human cadaveric heads are perfect for learning cerebrovascular anatomy, surgical approaches, and anatomy-related limitations of the operative field during a bypass procedure. However, fixed brain tissue and vessels have very different mechanical properties compared with living tissues. We believe that extra time and effort spent on the dissection of fixed cadaveric heads is inappropriate for the regular practice of microvascular bypass because of the abundance of more readily available tissue models. Such head models are more relevant for skill-oriented whole-procedure simulation. Several cadaveric head models with pressurized vessels and lightly fixed brains have been described for use in practical courses on cerebrovascular surgery.[6,7,8,9]

Human Placenta

Human placenta is a good source of small vessels for microsurgical practice. The human placenta has an oval shape with a diameter of 16 to 20 cm, a thickness of 2 to 3 cm, and weight of 500 to 600 g. The fetal surface of the placenta is covered with two closely adherent membranes, the chorion and amnion, which are similar to the arachnoid membrane and contain many vessels with diameters ranging from 1 to 6 mm. After approval is received from the local ethics committee, a placenta can be successfully used for microsurgical training (▶ Fig. 8.2).[10,11,12]

To prepare a placenta for use in microsurgical training, the student should remove the fetal allantoic sac and cut the umbilical cord, leaving a stump of about 5 cm length for insertion of the catheters for flushing the vascular beds and for pressurized infusion. The outer surface of the placenta then should be

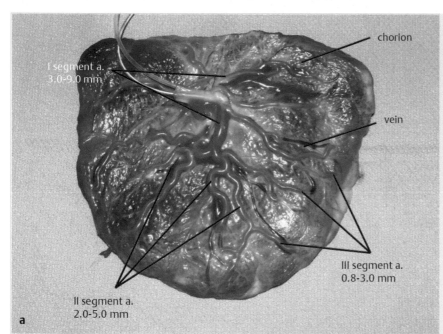

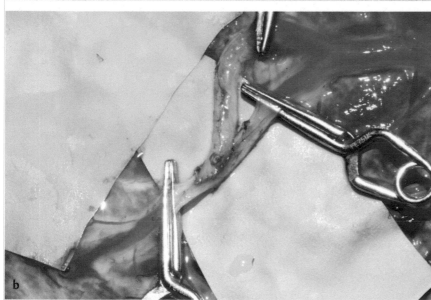

Fig. 8.2 Anastomosis training in a human placenta model. **(a)** Placenta prepared and connected to an infusion pump with colored solution for microsurgical training. **(b)** End-to-side anastomosis of 1-mm-diameter vessels. (Fig. 8.2a is reproduced with permission from Belykh E, Lei T, et al. Low-flow and high-flow neurosurgical bypass and anastomosis training models using human and bovine placental vessels: histological analysis and validation study. J Neurosurg. 2016;125(4):915–928.)

cleaned from blood products using tap water. Infusion of the cannulated umbilical cord arteries and veins with water or normal saline using a 50 mL syringe washes the blood clots from the vasculature. Cleaned placentas may be stored dry in a closed container under refrigeration (about 4 °C), but not frozen, for approximately 1 week during the training and then appropriately discarded.[10] We have attempted to store the placentas in isotonic solution, but we found that they are better preserved when stored without any solution.

Other Animal Material

Vessels for use in training can also be acquired from other animal species, including sheep heads and brains,[13] bovine placenta,[14] bovine heads,[15] and others. All of these models are a good source of fresh biological tissue that may be used for practicing microdissection and vessel suturing and handling skills. The common limitations of such models include the risk of infectious diseases and the need for special resources and logistics for acquisition, cleaning, storage, and disposal of biological materials.

8.2 Practice Schedule

8.2.1 When to Start Microsurgical Practice

Microsurgical training should begin as early as possible and include theoretical and practical courses. These courses should be divided into general and specialized training. General training is not dependent on the surgical specialization of a trainee and consists of learning laboratory animal care, anesthesia, microsurgical dissection, and suturing on synthetic and real tissue models. After learning these techniques, the curriculum should be directed toward learning specialized skills that are germane to the specific clinical goals of the trainee. Specialized training is conducted to gain proficiency in microsurgical techniques. The learning of difficult or specific skills and techniques is conducted purposefully to meet the requirements of a particular subspecialization or operation that the surgeon expects to perform.

8.2.2 Regularity

The educational process is most productive when the training sessions occur regularly and are of an appropriate duration. Training sessions should not be too short (shorter than 1 hour) or too long (longer than 4 hours), because fatigue will prevent optimal skill development. The most favorable duration for a dedicated session is 1 to 3 hours, with short rest periods every 40 minutes, or as necessary. The optimal time for practice is summer or holiday seasons when staff neurosurgeons take vacations and the volume of cases decreases. Many short courses offer basic 2-day microsurgical training. However, we believe that such training is less effective than ongoing, periodic training that occurs over a long period, despite the financial and logistical attractiveness of the shorter programs.

After 2 hours of working with a surgical microscope, a trainee may have difficulty with visual accommodation, which decreases the ability to focus, making training less effective. Additionally, microsurgery is full of details and subtleties that must be ingrained into habits, which are difficult to learn in such a short training period.

Approaches to microneurosurgical training schedules vary by nation, institution, and mentor. Good examples are neurosurgery departments and laboratories at universities in Kyoto, Fujita, and Fukui (Japan), where students and neurosurgery residents undergo rigorous and continuous training to master the basics of microsurgical training. The residents attend 2 classes of basic dry microsurgical training and practice 2 or 3 times per week in the laboratory over the course of their 7-year neurosurgical residency. Attending physicians and professors have free access to the laboratory and may also maintain their skills with regular exercises in addition to clinical practice.

8.2.3 Sample Structure of Microsurgical Training

The training begins with introductory lectures on the microsurgical tools and equipment (Chapters 1 and 2) and then 4 to 6 hours of dry training practice on knot tying and instrument handling (Chapter 3). The next 2 days are devoted to learning principles of work with laboratory animals, anesthesia, surgical approaches, and simple vascular anastomoses on a tissue model (Chapters 4 and 5). The following days are aimed to secure acquired skills and study more complex anastomoses on smaller arteries, veins, and in a deep operative field (Chapters 6 and 7).

Microsurgical training courses (Chapters 4–7) should be set at least annually and be performed along with cadaveric courses on neurosurgical anatomy and procedural simulation on computer virtual reality models. The dry training (Chapter 3) is then regularly used as a tool for rehearsal before an operation and to maintain microsurgical suturing skills. Finally, the microsurgical skills are refined in the operating room during real surgeries.

8.2.4 How to Get Involved

Training time goes by fast, and there is never enough time for regular training and practice in the laboratory. Several approaches may help the trainee to stay on schedule. If you want to pursue a career in cerebrovascular surgery, one good option is to seek an opportunity to collaborate with colleagues in the research department and to ask if you can work on a project that involves vascular surgery in rodents, such as arterial anastomoses or transplantations. Such research would result in the accumulation of necessary manual skills over time.

Trainees should practice microsurgery using the operative microscope whenever possible to develop the skills required for work under high magnification. Suturing the dura mater and closing wounds will initially take a long time under the microscope. As microsurgery skills are acquired, these procedures can be performed more quickly and with better precision and accuracy while the trainee's comfort with working with the operative microscope improves significantly.[16] Participate in advanced training courses on a regular basis, at least once per year. These practices are unique opportunities to go beyond the usual intraoperative scenarios and try new techniques.

Dry microsurgical training should be easily accessible in the resident's room. It should not take longer than moving a chair and turning on the light of the microscope to start a knot-tying practice session. The deliberate and focused practice of knotting techniques on a regular basis allows the student to sustain and advance their bypass skills. This practice may be performed every day even at home as off-the-job training.[17]

8.2.5 Training after Performing Bypass on a Patient

After 2 or more weeks of general training, the trainees should be ready to apply their acquired skills in clinical practice. However, students should remember that Dr. Yaşargil, esteemed for pioneering microneurosurgery, spent about a year in the laboratory practicing microsurgical bypasses performed on dozens of animals before he attempted his first microvascular extracranial-intracranial anastomosis on a patient.

Microsurgical training should not stop after the beginning of clinical application of a bypass. As in professional sports, athletes do not stop practicing their sport but intensify their practices. Beginning the clinical practice of bypass should encourage the surgeon to continue microsurgical training and seek opportunities to refine specific skills.

The mistakes of microsurgery can be rectified in most cases. However, such resolution is likely to be imperfect, possibly leading to unfavorable outcomes. An increase in the rates of bleeding, ischemia, and tissue necrosis can easily result. In the National Cardiovascular Center, in Kyoto, Japan, a neurosurgeon is only allowed to perform bypasses on patients after performing 100 successful bypasses on animals. Since vasospasm may easily develop in delicate small vessels, the result of microsurgical intervention must be interpreted as "all or nothing." It must be perfect. In most areas of medicine, the trend has been to blame systems for errors, not individuals. Although we might endorse this trend in most areas of medicine, the last time the system can intervene for the patient is in qualifying the surgeon. After that, the surgeon must assume the mantle of responsibility with appropriate preparation and humility.

8.3 Assessment of Microsurgical Performance and Skills

Current developments in simulation medicine require valid measures for the performance of basic surgical techniques and skills. These scales are important for senior colleagues and mentors to assess trainee improvements and for well-trained surgeons to know the training requirements for self-assess-

ment. Such objective measurements may contribute to a weighted decision for assigning assistance on a case or granting allowance for self-performance. Video recording of surgery and training is very helpful and is recommended for this purpose.

Performance scales are also useful in the development of scientific projects and the assessment of simulation models. The most reliable surgical scale is the Objective Structured Assessment of Technical Skills (OSATS), which has been used by the University of Toronto since the 1990s.[18] Based on this scale, a microsurgically relevant assessment scale was developed (▶ Table 8.1).[19] This scale is a reliable and valid scale that may be used for the assessment of microanastomosis performance. Another scale specifically aimed to assess aneurysm dissection and clipping may also be used to assess residents' and fellows' performance on experimental simulation models of cerebral aneurysm surgery (▶ Table 8.2). Virtual reality simulators are now very common for laparoscopy and robotic surgery training, and most of them include computer performance metrics.

Table 8.1 Northwestern Objective Microanastomosis Assessment Tool (NOMAT).[a]

Item	Poor performance	Moderate performance	High performance
I. Operator positioning and posture	Hunched back, twisted wrists, shrugged shoulders, wide range of movements.	Good posture and positioning at first but deteriorates by the end of the procedure. Rarely makes wide-ranging movements.	Optimally ergonomic and relaxed posture, with economy of movements. Movement is confined to the wrists and fingers.
II. Use of the surgical microscope	Readjusts positioning, focus, and working distance frequently, frequently out of focus or using a magnification level that impedes proper field navigation. Moves the surgical setting instead of navigating it with the scope.	Focused most of the time but readjusts at multiple instances, familiar with the use of the microscope but not yet proficient.	Optimizes zoom, focus, and optical settings at the beginning of the task and adjusts only when needed.
III. Understanding of the surgical equipment	Repeatedly uses the wrong instrument for the task.	Uses the correct instrument for the task most of the time, quickly switches to the correct instrument after a mistake.	Perfect matching of instruments and tasks. Knows the instruments well, and chooses according to the surgical need.
IV. Handling of the surgical instruments	Repeatedly makes tentative or awkward moves with instruments.	Competent use of instruments, although occasionally appears stiff and awkward.	Fluid moves with instruments, with no awkwardness.
V. Vessel handling and respect for tissue	Frequently damages the vessel by inappropriate use of force, with perforation or tearing of the wall. Tearing of the vessel by inappropriate needle or instrument handling or during knot tying.	Acceptable/occasional accidental damage that does not affect the structural integrity of the vessel but could theoretically thrombosis and cause intimal damage. Rough movements at the anastomotic line during knot tying.	Vessel almost intact at the end of the procedure. Absence of movements that may promote intimal endothelial damage or thrombosis. High handling proficiency.
VI. Needle handling and care	Irreparable damage to the needle requiring a new suture thread to complete the anastomosis.	The needle is moderately damaged and deformed but still functional.	The needle is undamaged and un-deformed at the end of the procedure.
VII. Needle bite uniformity	Needle bites are very uneven between the two edges of the anastomosis. Needle bites are very irregular from suture point to suture point.	Approximately 50% of needle bites are even and regular.	All needle bites are even and regular.
VIII. Spacing of the sutures	Constant irregular intervals. Suboptimal number of suture points is used to complete the anastomosis (more or less than 10-12 for 3 mm and 6-8 for 1 mm).	>50% of intervals are equal and regular, but a suboptimal number of suture points is used to complete the anastomosis (more or less than 10-12 for 3 mm and 6-8 for 1 mm).	Intervals are equal. The number of suture points is appropriate for the vessel size (10-12 for 3 mm and 6-8 for 1 mm).
IX. Knot-tying	Knots are too loose and could potentially be undone. Knots are tight enough to cut through or shred the vessel. Wastes a lot of thread and requires multiple (>3 total) new suture threads to finish the anastomosis.	Acceptable knot quality but uneven or irregular. The sutures are cut at an inappropriate length. Requires 1 additional suture thread to finish the anastomosis.	Perfect square knots with good knot strength and tension. Appropriate suture length. Finished the entire anastomosis using only one suture thread.

Table 8.1 continued

Item	Poor performance	Moderate performance	High performance
X. Microsurgical efficiency with the needle	Many unnecessary moves. Multiple attempts needed to grasp the needle. Multiple passes required to successfully bite the tissue. Loses the needle frequently in the surgical field.	Few unnecessary moves. Few attempts to successfully grasp the needle. Few passes are required to successfully bite the tissue.	No wasted moves, grasps only once. Economy of movement and efficiency. Mostly single attempts/passes to successfully bite the tissue.
XI. Microsurgical efficiency with knot tying	Many unnecessary moves. Multiple attempts needed to grasp the suture and tie the knot. Multiple suture breaks or kinks from excessive force.	Few unnecessary moves. Few attempts to successfully grasp the suture. Minimal breaks that do not impede knot tying.	No wasted moves. Economy of movement and efficiency. Mostly single attempts/passes to successfully tie a knot.
XII. Evaluation of the completed anastomosis - Off-pump	Severe vessel kinking, angulation, or torsion. Vessel completely deformed. Did not complete the anastomosis.	No vascular torsion. Mild vessel kinking.	Good anastomotic line. Anastomosis predicted to be functional.
XIII. Evaluation of the completed anastomosis - On-pump	Jet of fluid originating from between adjacent sutures. Profuse oozing without specific focal point. Vessel sewn shut. No flow.	Moderate oozing without specific focal points.	Slight oozing originating mostly from needle entry and exit points that would be controlled in vivo by the application of cotton.
XIV. Evaluation of the completed anastomosis - Examination of the lumen	>70% lumen stenosis, back wall caught by a suture point.	10 to 50% lumen stenosis. Overlapping vessel edges with minimal compromise. Free back wall.	No considerable stenosis that would restrict the vessel and blood flow.

[a]Items were scored on a scale from 1 to 5, where 1 is poor performance and 5 is high performance. Revised with permission from El Ahmadieh TY, Aoun SG, El Tecle NE, et al. A didactic and hands-on module enhances resident microsurgical knowledge and technical skill. Neurosurgery. 2013;73 Suppl 1:51-56.

Table 8.2 Objective Structured Assessment of Aneurysm Clipping Skills (OSACS).[a]

Item	Poor performance	Moderate performance	High performance
Operator positioning and posture	Hunched back, twisted wrists, shrugged shoulders, wide range of movements	Good posture and positioning at first but deteriorates by the end of the procedure, rarely makes wide-range movements	Optimally ergonomic and relaxed posture; economy of movements
Use of the surgical microscope	Readjusts positioning, focus, and working distance frequently, frequently out of focus or using a magnification level that impedes proper field navigation	Focused most of the time but readjusts at multiple instances, familiar with the use of the microscope but not yet proficient	Optimizes zoom, focus, and optical settings at the beginning of the task and adjusts only when needed
Knowledge of instruments	Repetitively uses the wrong instrument for the task	Uses the correct instrument for the task most of the time, quickly switches to the correct instrument after a mistake	Perfect matching of instruments and tasks at hand, knows the instruments well and chooses according to the surgical need
Instrument handling	Repeatedly makes tentative or awkward moves with instruments	Competent use of instruments, although occasionally appears stiff and awkward	Fluid moves with instruments and no awkwardness
Time and motion	Many unnecessary moves	Efficient time and motion but some unnecessary moves	Economy of movement and maximum efficiency
Time flow of operation and forward planning	Frequently stops operating or needs to discuss next move	Demonstrates ability for forward planning with steady progression of operative procedure	Obviously planned course of operation with effortless flow from one move to the next
Quality of aneurysm clipping	Poor technique, parent vessel compromise or insufficient clipping	Moderately good technique, parent vessel is patent or slightly stenosed, complete exclusion of aneurysm	Excellent technique, optimal clip position, aneurysm excluded from flow, no parent artery compromise
Respect for tissue	Often uses unnecessary force on tissue or causes damage by inappropriate use of instruments	Careful handling of tissue but occasionally causes inadvertent damage	Consistently handles tissue appropriately with minimal damage
Quality of dissection	Poor technique, frequent damage of vessels, insufficient aneurysm exposure	Moderately good technique of dissection in proximity to the vessels with acceptable or occasional accidental damage that does not affect the structural integrity of the vessel, adequate exposure of the aneurysm and parent vessels	Excellent technique of sharp and blind dissection, uninjured vessels, adequate and sufficient exposure of the aneurysm and parent vessels

[a]Items were scored on a scale from 1 to 5, where 1 is poor performance and 5 is high performance. Used with permission from Belykh E, Miller EJ, Lei T, et al. Face, content, and construct validity of an aneurysm clipping model using human placenta. World Neurosurg. 2017;105:952-960.

However, such virtual reality simulators have yet to become available for microvascular practice.[20]

Sidebar

Short training sessions are enough to acquire microsurgical skills, but these sessions must be done regularly. Make 10 sutures on gauze forming a cross with the left and right hands daily. Vary the training exercises from time to time to create a challenge (in the operating room, the conditions are not ideal). Simulate manipulations in a deep surgical wound, practice suturing on gauze in different directions, make anastomoses on elastic tubes, and remember to train on biological tissues (wet training).

References

[1] Olabe J, Olabe J. Microsurgical training on an in vitro chicken wing infusion model. Surg Neurol; 72(6):695–699

[2] Hino A. Training in microvascular surgery using a chicken wing artery. Neurosurgery; 52(6):1495–1497, discussion 1497–1498

[3] Abla AA, Uschold T, Preul MC, Zabramski JM. Comparative use of turkey and chicken wing brachial artery models for microvascular anastomosis training. J Neurosurg; 115(6):1231–1235

[4] Colpan ME, Slavin KV, Amin-Hanjani S, Calderon-Arnuphi M, Charbel FT. Microvascular anastomosis training model based on a Turkey neck with perfused arteries. Neurosurgery; 62(5) Suppl 2:ONS407–ONS410, discussion ONS410–ONS411

[5] Olabe J, Olabe J, Sancho V. Human cadaver brain infusion model for neurosurgical training. Surg Neurol; 72(6):700–702

[6] Olabe J, Olabe J, Roda JM, Sancho V. Human cadaver brain infusion skull model for neurosurgical training. Surg Neurol Int; 2:54

[7] Russin JJ, Mack WJ, Carey JN, Minneti M, Giannotta SL. Simulation of a high-flow extracranial-intracranial bypass using a radial artery graft in a novel fresh tissue model. Neurosurgery; 71(2) Suppl Operative:ons315–ons319, discussion 319–320

[8] Aboud E, Aboud G, Al-Mefty O, et al. "Live cadavers" for training in the management of intraoperative aneurysmal rupture. J Neurosurg; 123(5):1339–1346

[9] Aboud E, Al-Mefty O, Yaşargil MG. New laboratory model for neurosurgical training that simulates live surgery. J Neurosurg; 97(6):1367–1372

[10] Oliveira Magaldi M, Nicolato A, Godinho JV, et al. Human placenta aneurysm model for training neurosurgeons in vascular microsurgery. Neurosurgery; 10 Suppl 4:592–600, discussion 600–601

[11] Ayoubi S, Ward P, Naik S, Sankaran M. The use of placenta in a microvascular exercise. Neurosurgery; 30(2):252–254

[12] Romero FR, Fernandes ST, Chaddad-Neto F, Ramos JG, Campos JM, Oliveira Ed. Microsurgical techniques using human placenta. Arq Neuropsiquiatr; 66(4):876–878

[13] Hamamcioglu MK, Hicdonmez T, Tiryaki M, Cobanoglu S. A laboratory training model in fresh cadaveric sheep brain for microneurosurgical dissection of cranial nerves in posterior fossa. Br J Neurosurg; 22(6):769–771

[14] Belykh EG, Lei T, Oliveira MM, et al. Carotid endarterectomy surgical simulation model using a bovine placenta vessel. Neurosurgery; 77(5):825–829, discussion 829–830

[15] Hicdonmez T, Hamamcioglu MK, Tiryaki M, Cukur Z, Cobanoglu S. Microneurosurgical training model in fresh cadaveric cow brain: a laboratory study simulating the approach to the circle of Willis. Surg Neurol; 66(1):100–104, discussion 104

[16] Kivelev J, Hernesniemi J. Four-fold benefit of wound closure under high magnification. Surg Neurol Int; 4:115

[17] Belykh E, Byvaltsev V. Off-the-job microsurgical training on dry models: Siberian experience. World Neurosurg; 82(1–2):20–24

[18] Reznick R, Regehr G, MacRae H, Martin J, McCulloch W. Testing technical skill via an innovative "bench station" examination. Am J Surg; 173(3):226–230

[19] Aoun SG, El Ahmadieh TY, El Tecle NE, et al. A pilot study to assess the construct and face validity of the Northwestern Objective Microanastomosis Assessment Tool. J Neurosurg; 123(1):103–109

[20] Helal-An-Nahiyan M, Farhin M, Lim G. Design and simulation of a training simulation of microvascular anastomosis with visual and haptic feedback. IJSRP; 5(8):1–4

9 Possible Bypass Errors

Evgenii Belykh and Peter Nakaji

Abstract

This chapter describes common pitfalls and mistakes that can be made during anastomosis practice. Learning about them early in your training can help you avoid them or compensate for them during actual surgery. Junior neurosurgeons, in particular, can benefit from learning how to prevent errors and how to cope with them when they do occur.

Keywords: bleeding, bypasses, complications, errors, failures, mistakes, occlusion, thrombosis

9.1 Possible Bypass Errors

We can all learn from our mistakes, particularly early in our training. By taking advantage of the opportunity to learn from our mistakes in the laboratory, we may be able to better avoid mistakes in our future clinical practice. One area of potential improvement is bypass errors.

Amin-Hanjani and Charbel[1] classified bypass errors into two main types: poor indications for bypass and technical errors with the bypass. They also defined three subtypes of technical errors: donor vessel problems, anastomosis problems, and outflow vessel problems.

Numerous common mistakes can occur during bypass procedures. Most of these mistakes are technical in nature and might be avoided through laboratory practice, which helps you to anticipate and circumvent such mistakes. Although a detailed analysis of clinical management guidelines, such as appropriate selection of treatment strategies, is beyond the scope of this manual, certain aspects of these guidelines are important to consider in order to preclude common mistakes that can be potentially devastating to the patient.

9.2 Patient–Treatment Mismatch

Selecting bypass surgery for a patient who is not a suitable candidate for such treatment is the first mistake that should be avoided. Outcomes for extracranial-intracranial (EC-IC) bypasses from the Carotid Occlusion Surgery Study[2] and the Japanese EC-IC Bypass Trial[3] showed the EC-IC bypass to be inferior to the best medical treatment for intracranial ischemic disease, thus greatly reducing indications for this procedure. Clearly, even a technically excellent bypass can fail to benefit patients who were not carefully selected.

Mistiming the bypass for the patient, such as by rushing to perform it, can also be problematic. Enough time should be allowed before surgery to control modifiable risk factors and to adjust the patient's blood coagulation and platelet profile. Patients are usually given low-dose aspirin (81–100 mg/day) before a bypass and full-dose aspirin (325 mg/day) after the bypass. To overcome aspirin resistance, you should run the aspirin response test and adjust the aspirin dosage as needed.[4] A slight increase in bleeding during surgery as a result of aspirin use is preferable to a bypass clot, which can lead to a stroke.

9.3 Operating Room Environment and Operative Team

Extra supplies should be readily available during an anastomosis, as not having them on hand can present problems. All extra microneurosurgery tools that compose the bypass instrument set (microsurgical forceps, scissors, clips, sutures, and bipolar forceps) should be prepared for use before commencing the procedure. Bipolar coagulation power settings should be adjusted to a low setting after switching to the microsurgical bipolar forceps and before starting to coagulate branches on a small recipient cortical artery.

In addition to requiring the right equipment and backup instruments, the bypass procedure also requires a well-trained team and good teamwork. Despite the observation or participation of medical students, residents, and other trainees, the operating room is not the best place to teach bypass workflow, which instead should be practiced in the laboratory.

The operating room setup should offer the surgeon the optimal position and a comfortable posture, because poor posture can result in excessive tremor, which can undermine the skill set of any surgeon (Video 9.1).

9.4 Anesthesia-Related Issues

Errors in blood pressure management can have a huge effect on the degree of cerebral perfusion. Decreasing blood pressure during the operation to a level below what is typical for a particular patient may cause an infarction either near to or distant from the bypass location. The blood pressure levels of patients should be strictly maintained at their awake blood pressure levels while they are under general anesthesia during surgery.

It is important to be aware of several key areas where anesthesia-related mistakes can occur. Communication with the anesthesiologist is therefore key. First, hyperventilation should be avoided during bypass surgery. Second, alpha-adrenergic agonists are not recommended because of their vasoconstrictive effects. Third, if the brain is bulging, mannitol should be administered instead of hyperventilation, and the anesthesia can be deepened by increasing the propofol dose under tight blood pressure control. Fourth, during the temporary clipping and while anastomosis is being performed, barbiturates or propofol should be used routinely for burst suppression under electroencephalogram monitoring.

9.5 Donor Vessel

There are several mistakes that can occur during the dissection of a donor vessel. The first potential mistake involves confusing the superficial temporal artery with the superficial temporal vein. To avoid this error, keep in mind that the vein is usually straight, blue, and thin, whereas the artery is usually more curved, white, and pulsatile. A second possible mistake is to mishandle the donor vessel so as to damage it, to allow it to dry out, or to cause it to go into spasm. This mistake can be avoided by keeping the donor vessel or graft moist and warm, which will prevent it from spasming. The heat from newer microscopes can quickly dry out a donor vessel, so be sure to continuously irrigate the vessel. If the vessel does spasm, you can abort the spasming by rinsing it with the papaverine, nicardipine, milrinone, or a local anesthetic.

The occipital artery takes longer to dissect than the superficial temporal artery. Therefore, you should determine beforehand whether the occipital artery will be considered as a donor and should spend precious time on its dissection only after this decision is made.

Scalp necrosis and wound infection after decreasing the scalp blood supply by dissecting and redirecting the temporal or occipital artery is another concern. The reported incidence of wound infection or necrosis associated with bypass procedures varies between 0.7 and 21.4%, and this incidence is considered to be higher than that associated with craniotomies without skin vessel harvesting.[5,6,7,8] The major factors predisposing to wound problems include harvesting of both branches of the superficial temporal artery, diabetes, and atherosclerosis obliterans.[7,8] Other suggested factors include traumatic handling of the tissue edge, damage to the galeal vessels, and marginal location of the harvested vessel within the flap.[8] Although studies have not had enough statistical power to show the benefit of a particular incision shape, such as straight skin incision over flaps, in preventing wound complications,[7] thoughtful and careful skin incision planning is important to avoid such complications.

A pedunculated donor vessel should be large enough (> 1 mm in diameter) to provide adequate flow. In many cases where direct bypass was found to be technically impossible, it was due to an occluded, atretic, or small donor vessel.[5] In cases in which there is a small donor vessel, the bypass strategy can be adjusted in several ways: indirect bypass could be used, the donor vessel could be cut proximally (where it is larger) and an interposition graft could be used, or an alternative donor vessel, such as the maxillary artery, could be used.[5,9]

9.6 Craniotomy

The most important mistake to avoid in performing a craniotomy is damaging the donor vessel with the drill. To avoid this mistake, place a Farabeuf retractor or Penfield dissector between the craniotome blade and the vessel to protect the soft tissues from being accidentally damaged by the drill. Do not place the donor vessel under a cottonoid patty or gauze, because this material could be caught by the drill. Avoid using a fishhook retractor or another compressive type of retractor on the donor vessel. You can also perform a larger dissection at the proximal and distal ends of the vessel from the galea, so that the vessel can be retracted farther away from the trajectory of the drill foot plate.

9.7 Choosing a Recipient Vessel

In selecting a recipient vessel for a bypass, you should not suture a smaller donor vessel to a larger recipient vessel—even when circulation is compromised—because it will not result in good blood flow. This mistake can be avoided by selecting a recipient vessel that is the same size as or smaller than the donor vessel. The pressure in large intracranial vessels is usually high, and a narrow donor vessel could result in slow flow at the anastomosis. Measuring the blood flow accurately is therefore important for assessing and matching blood flow demand and supply.[1]

9.8 Operative Field

To avoid problems in the operative field, it should be cleaned, cleaned, and cleaned again. Trying to work in a dirty or bloody operative field is a common mistake that can complicate the bypass. Do not hesitate to spend extra time to make the operative field perfectly clean before attempting a bypass, including making sure that the microsuction device is working well. Even when you do everything else perfectly, patient bleeding can severely obscure the view and hamper your every movement. It is often best to use an extra rubber dam around the vessel, so that, when you are sewing, the sutures fall on a clean surface rather than stick to brain, muscle, or clotted blood.

9.9 Instruments

Neglecting the condition of the instruments that will be used to perform a procedure can undermine even the most well-practiced microsurgical skill. Even the most meticulous attempt to tailor the vessels for the anastomosis will fail if your microscissors are damaged or your microsurgical forceps are bent. Using only high-quality bypass scissors and the sharpest brand-new blades will enable you to successfully trim the donor and recipient vessels to achieve perfectly matching fish-mouth incisions. Check microneurosurgical instruments thoroughly before every surgical procedure, and send them immediately for repair if necessary, especially if you must use a shared operating room instrument set. Most neurosurgeons have their own set of instruments for bypass procedures. If you do carry your own instruments, make sure that they are sterilized and are in excellent condition before and after every procedure.

9.10 Vessel Preparation

A common mistake in vessel preparation is not being precise enough when matching the sizes of the openings in the donor and recipient vessels. Any overlaps will complicate the suturing. If the size of the two vessels is a mismatch, then you will have to focus on using the whole length of the vessel to avoid creating a "dog-ear" at the end. Before starting to suture, take time to align the two openings perfectly (▶ Fig. 9.1).

Another scenario that can be problematic is when there is not enough room between the opening in the recipient vessel and the clip. Not having enough space to maneuver can complicate vessel rotation and suturing. Therefore, apply clips to the recipient vessel in such a way as to keep enough space for vessel rotation and suturing of the back wall.

For optimal results, an end-to-side anastomosis should be 2 to 2.5 times larger than the diameter of the recipient vessel. The anastomosis should not be the point of flow resistance. Even if the anastomosis is contracted, which is difficult to see, it should still be large enough to allow adequate flow.

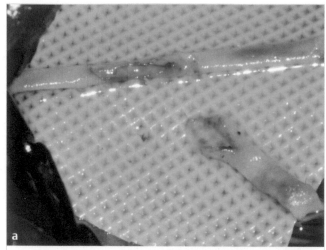

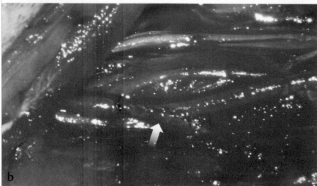

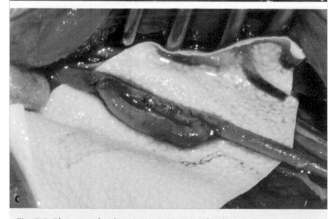

Fig. 9.1 Photographs demonstrating a vessel tailoring mistake. **(a)** The upper vessel is an example of a badly tailored recipient vessel with an incision that was made too large. **(b)** Stenosis (*arrow*) and thrombosis after anastomosis. **(c)** Microscopic view of the anastomosis shows stenosed vessel segment. A second anastomosis was performed proximally using the same vessels in an end-to-side fashion. Note that the blood flow bypasses the thrombosed segment through the functioning heel part of the first anastomosis.

If the backwall suturing is not possible from the outside of the vessel, it should be done from inside, similar to typical side-to-side anastomosis. In such a situation, a slightly larger anastomosis, optimally three times larger than the diameter of the recipient vessel, is more convenient than a smaller anastomosis, because it leaves more space for needle passes and suturing of the back wall.

Be careful to remove the temporary clips in the correct sequence to avoid air and microthrombi emboli. Distal clips should be removed first to allow back filling, followed by removal of the proximal clip and, finally, removal of the temporary clip on the donor vessel.

9.11 Running Suture

Another potential mistake that is easy to avoid is to start the ischemia time without first making sure that all other aspects of the procedure have advanced as far as possible and that everything else is prepared. For instance, you should put the heel and toe stitches on the donor vessel before occluding the recipient vessel to save time.

A common suturing mistake involves starting the first puncture from inside the vessel. Doing so leaves the tail of the suture in the lumen of the vessel, which requires one to start from the beginning (from outside) and costs time.

Another suturing mistake is to make the loops too tight at the beginning. To make perfect loops, keep them small, loose, and stack them at first. Then tighten them sequentially at the end. If you tighten the loops one by one as you make them, the adventitia is more likely to protrude into the lumen, which can promote thrombosis.

Failure to anticipate and preventively address difficult parts of the anastomosis, such as the heel area, is another potential suturing mistake. The most difficult sutures to make are usually those closer to the heel than to the toe, because such sutures are hidden somewhat by the donor artery. A suturing mistake, such as tearing the vessel wall, or persistent bleeding can often occur closer to the heel. Thus, sutures close to the heel should be done first, before vessel rotation is restricted by other sutures.

Be careful not to pierce the opposite wall when placing running sutures. Once you have completely finished one wall of the anastomosis, it is extremely difficult to repair running sutures. If you do pierce the opposite wall, repair of the running sutures will require release of the captured wall. In most cases, such a mistake eventually requires that the running suture be completely redone, because even if you cut and release the captured opposite wall from the suture loop, the extra suture length that is thereby released may loosen the whole suture line. If the released loop is not so large, it can be evenly redistributed through the whole suture line without compromising anastomosis patency. An additional interrupted suture can sometimes be placed and tied with a loose loop to restore the tension across the suture line. If the captive loop is cut, the neighboring stiches can be released to free up the suture ends, which can be tied with an additional "repair" running suture. However, such methods usually necessitate release of at least two loops in each direction (four loops total), which, in practical terms, may be no different from redoing the running suture.

Finally, it is a mistake to allow tangling of the loops during a running suture. Doing so can create a blocking suture when the needle is accidentally passed inside the preceding loop.

9.12 Knots and Thread

A common mistake with knots is to use too many. You will rarely encounter the need for more than three knots. Because nylon sutures are prone to breakage, another common mistake is to leave them bent, deformed, and broken within a knot, especially during a running suture. Your suture-handling technique should be developed enough to avoid thread damage. During actual surgery, you should be sure to use only needles and sutures that are in perfect condition (i.e., not bent). If the suture is damaged, it is better to replace it. However, during training, especially in the early stages, you should try to save as much of the suture as possible to make maximal use of every thread.

9.13 Interrupted Suture

When performing the end-to-end anastomosis, you should not apply the clips without considering how the vessel will rotate and possibly complicate continued suturing. The clips should be placed so that you can turn the clips over, rotating the vessel with them, to see and suture the back wall.

It is easy to become confused while suturing, pierce the vessel wall behind the one to which you are suturing with the needle, and capture the vessel wall with the suture, especially when trying to suture a collapsed vessel. Ideally, the vessel exposure and clip rotation should allow positioning of the vessel such that there is no "difficult" side of anastomosis. You should frequently double-check the stitches that have been placed to ensure that you have not accidentally grabbed the opposite wall.

Finally, it is a mistake to pass the needle in such a way that it takes in too much of the vessel wall or such that the knots, when tightened, are either too tight or too loose (▶ Fig. 9.2,

Video 9.2). Overly tight knots cause corrugation and stenosis and can result in the adventitia curling and protruding inside. At the opposite extreme, loose sutures may result in excess thread inside the vessel, which can lead to thrombosis or anastomosis leakage.

9.14 Grabbing the Vessel

Squeezing the vessel wall with the forceps can produce enough endothelial damage to result in thrombosis. Sometimes the angle at which you have to work does not allow the use of a counterpressure technique, so you have to grab the vessel edge with the forceps. When this is the case, you should grab the vessel carefully to ensure that anything that has been grabbed stays outside the lumen, at the wall edge where the suture is going to come through.

9.15 Bleeding

When bleeding occurs during the process of creating an anastomosis, it can be a mistake to allow too much clotting. Try to be patient and avoid using an excessive amount of hemostatic material or pressing too hard in trying to stop the bleeding. You have to be patient to press just hard enough to stop the bleeding without compressing the vessel. Probably the best hemostatic material is a crushed piece of muscle, which is less likely than other hemostatic materials to get inside the anastomosis. To stop the bleeding, you can also use a commercially available hemostat, such as Surgicel Nu-Knit (Ethicon US, LLC, Cincinnati,

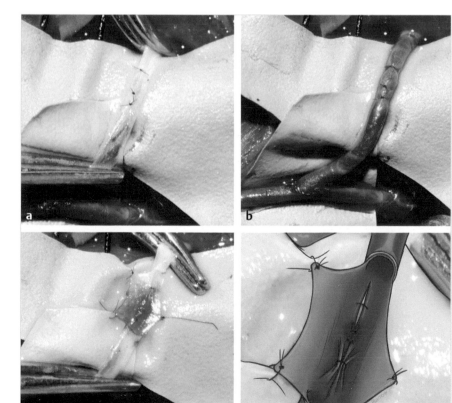

Fig. 9.2 Photographs and illustration demonstrating suturing mistakes. (a) Three sutures intentionally placed in an incorrect manner to demonstrate potential mistakes in closing the arteriotomy. The upper suture is too loose, the middle suture has adventitia protruding inside, and the lower suture is grabbing too much tissue, which creates folds and constrictions. (b) The defects caused by these three types of suturing mistakes are apparent when the blood flow is restored. (c) Intraoperative photograph and (d) artist's illustration of the inside of the vessel, which has been opened and stained with dye. Both (c) and (d) demonstrate the loose upper suture, the adventitia protruding inside the middle suture, and the constriction caused by the overreaching of the lower suture.

Ohio). Oftentimes, the actual bleeding is from a small branch of a donor vessel (e.g., the superior temporal artery or a radial artery) or a small branch of a cortical cerebral artery near the anastomosis. Irrigation with saline solution will reveal the source of the bleeding so that the bleeding can be addressed.

9.16 Assessing Flow

Assessing the flow too soon after completing the anastomosis can sometimes result in false-positive findings. Wait 10 to 15 minutes before making a final judgment to decrease the likelihood of missing thrombosis. Then look not only for flow but also to make sure that there is no back flow or slow flow that does not fill the vessel right away. If back flow is detected or if the flow does not fill the vessel immediately, the reason for the failure should be determined, and the procedure will need to be performed again.

9.17 Wound Closure

Mistakes in closing the surgical wound include making the closure too loose, stabbing the donor vessel, and underestimating the need for hemostasis and drainage. Although trying to achieve watertight closure of the dura is difficult due to penetrating the donor vessel, tight closure of the galea and subcutaneous skin layers is important to prevent a cerebrospinal fluid leak. During closure, you should take special care not to stab the donor vessel. You should also pay meticulous attention to hemostasis and drainage, because the patient will be administered a postoperative regimen of antiplatelets after undergoing EC-IC bypass. In addition, special care should be taken to evenly distribute skin tension during closure to avoid ischemic skin necrosis.

9.18 Postoperative Period

Several aspects of patient care should be addressed in the postoperative period. It can be a mistake to use a compressive dressing on patients immediately after bypass surgery or even to allow them to wear their eyeglasses too soon. You should document these restrictions in your postoperative notes. Tissues are especially swollen after the operation and can compress a vessel against eyeglass frames or bandages.

Postoperative blood pressure should be closely monitored and aggressively managed to avoid letting it get too low or too high. After even a standard uncomplicated case, patients should be placed under close observation for 48 hours. Patients are given aspirin at a dosage of 325 mg/day after surgery for the first year and are screened for aspirin sensitivity in the first few weeks after initiating the regimen. After 1 year, patients may continue to receive 325 mg/day, or the regimen may be adjusted to 81 mg/day according to their medical needs or the preference of their primary care provider.

9.19 Conclusion

By learning about many areas in which mistakes can potentially occur and by practicing how to respond to such mistakes in the laboratory, you will be better prepared to deal with these situations when they occur in the operating suite. Importantly, you can also learn how to anticipate difficulties and avoid them.

References

[1] Amin-Hanjani S, Charbel FT. Flow-assisted surgical technique in cerebrovascular surgery. Surg Neurol; 68 Suppl 1:S4–S11

[2] Powers WJ, Clarke WR, Grubb RL , Jr, Videen TO, Adams HP , Jr, Derdeyn CP, COSS Investigators. Extracranial-intracranial bypass surgery for stroke prevention in hemodynamic cerebral ischemia: the Carotid Occlusion Surgery Study randomized trial. JAMA; 306(18):1983–1992

[3] Ogasawara K, Ogawa A. [JET study (Japanese EC-IC Bypass Trial)]. Nihon Rinsho; 64 Suppl 7:524–527

[4] Jussen D, Horn P, Vajkoczy P. Aspirin resistance in patients with hemodynamic cerebral ischemia undergoing extracranial-intracranial bypass surgery. Cerebrovasc Dis; 35(4):355–362

[5] Mesiwala AH, Sviri G, Fatemi N, Britz GW, Newell DW. Long-term outcome of superficial temporal artery-middle cerebral artery bypass for patients with moyamoya disease in the US. Neurosurg Focus; 24(2):E15

[6] Abla AA, Gandhoke G, Clark JC, et al. Surgical outcomes for moyamoya angiopathy at Barrow Neurological Institute with comparison of adult indirect encephaloduroarteriosynangiosis bypass, adult direct superficial temporal artery-to-middle cerebral artery bypass, and pediatric bypass: 154 revascularization surgeries in 140 affected hemispheres. Neurosurgery; 73(3):430–439

[7] Katsuta T, Inoue T, Arakawa S, Uda K. Cutaneous necrosis after superficial temporal artery-to-middle cerebral artery anastomosis: is it predictable or avoidable? Neurosurgery; 49(4):879–882, discussion 882–884

[8] Takanari K, Araki Y, Okamoto S, et al. Operative wound-related complications after cranial revascularization surgeries. J Neurosurg; 123(5):1145–1150

[9] Yağmurlu K, Kalani MYS, Martirosyan NL, et al. Maxillary artery to middle cerebral artery bypass: a novel technique for exposure of the maxillary artery. World Neurosurg; 100:540–550

10 Translation of Laboratory Skills: Indications for Bypass in Neurosurgery

Evgenii Belykh, M. Yashar S. Kalani, Vadim A. Byvaltsev, and Peter Nakaji

Abstract

This chapter is devoted to the description of basic clinical concepts related to vascular bypass procedures. In this chapter, we describe the terminology related to bypass procedures that is used in neurosurgery. We also describe the classification of bypasses, and we systematically describe a wide spectrum of possible surgical solutions when choosing a bypass procedure. Surgical techniques of low-flow and high-flow extracranial-intracranial bypasses are also described.

Keywords: bypass, classification, extracranial-intracranial bypass, flow augmentation, high flow, in situ reconstruction, low flow, middle cerebral artery bypass, superficial temporal artery bypass

10.1 Introduction

This chapter describes the basic techniques of extracranial-intracranial (EC-IC) bypass operations. The next chapter, *Case Examples of Cerebrovascular Bypass*, focuses on disease-specific considerations.

10.2 Types of Bypass

To treat ischemia or to replace blood flow when a vessel needs to be sacrificed, direct, indirect, or combined bypass procedures can be performed to produce collateral blood flow. Direct bypass reroutes blood flow from a donor artery to a recipient artery through the anastomosis. The most common example is anastomosing an extracranial vessel with an intracranial vessel. While performing a direct bypass, it is necessary to temporarily occlude the recipient cerebral artery. It has been shown that such occlusion of the middle cerebral artery (MCA) during anastomosis of the superficial temporal artery (STA) to the MCA does not compromise cerebral metabolic or electrical activity in most patients.[1] Direct anastomosis provides immediate blood flow, and its patency can be measured intraoperatively by Doppler, fluorescence video-angiography (indocyanine green angiography), or digital subtraction angiography. Indirect revascularization artificially optimizes conditions for the induction of neovascularization by attaching different types of tissues to the brain surface. The donor tissues can be dura, muscle, or omentum, although the use of omentum is rare.

10.2.1 General Principles of Direct Neurosurgical Bypass Procedures

Bypass surgery has numerous nuances and employs various operative techniques. In this section, we will summarize general principles of bypass surgeries. We will systematically describe the wide spectrum of available options to consider when tailoring the surgical strategy for each individual patient's anatomy and lesion, discuss the techniques for bypass in vascular reconstruction, and identify different operative strategies for bypass procedures.

Aim of Bypass

In cases of brain ischemia, bypass strategies aim to support a hemodynamically compromised watershed and to reverse ischemia or prevent its further progression (▶ Fig. 10.1). Thus, the term *blood flow augmentation* is used to classify this type of bypass.[2,3] In most cases of aneurysm trapping, the goal of bypass is to replace the preexisting normal blood flow through the parent artery and its distal branches; therefore, the term *blood flow replacement* is used.[4] Indications for flow replacement bypass are tumors (benign and malignant), vascular lesions (giant aneurysms and dural arteriovenous fistulas), and traumatic or iatrogenic vascular injuries. In complicated aneurysms, the preference between the terms blood flow augmentation and blood flow replacement is based on the estimated flow demand. Both low- and high-flow grafts are applicable, but the latter is preferable because it can carry almost the same blood flow as the internal carotid artery (ICA).

Volume of Blood Flow

The volume of blood flow is used to classify reconstructive bypass procedures (▶ Fig. 10.2). Historically, bypasses have been classified as low flow or high flow, and this definition is still widely used. *Low-flow* bypasses usually use an STA-MCA bypass, and *high-flow* bypasses usually use bypasses from the carotid arteries in the neck to intracranial arteries using vascular grafts, such as radial artery grafts or saphenous vein grafts.[5,6,7] Technically, when describing a bypass, the terms low- and high-flow refer to the grafts: low-flow vessel grafts have a flow rate of 20 to 70 mL/min,[8] intermediate-flow vessels have a flow rate of 60 to 100 mL/min, and high-flow vessels have a flow rate of 100 mL/min or greater.[9] However, in many reported series, the flow was not measured directly. Mohit et al[10] classified patients as having

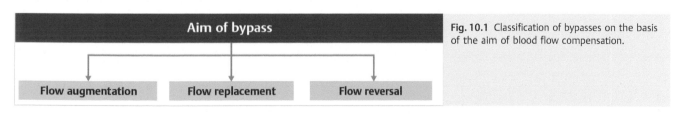

Fig. 10.1 Classification of bypasses on the basis of the aim of blood flow compensation.

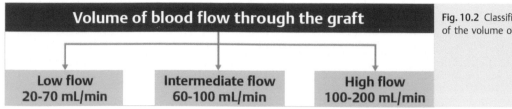

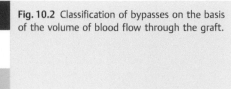

Fig. 10.2 Classification of bypasses on the basis of the volume of blood flow through the graft.

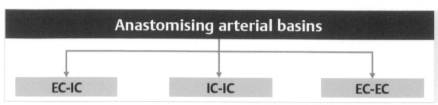

Fig. 10.3 Classification of bypasses on the basis of the anastomosing arterial basins. Abbreviations: EC-IC, extracranial-intracranial; IC-IC, intracranial-intracranial; EC-EC, extracranial-extracranial.

high-flow bypass when a radial artery graft or saphenous vein graft was used; patients were classified as having low-flow bypass when they underwent other bypass procedures, including STA-MCA bypass, A3-A3 bypass, reimplantation, primary repair, posterior inferior cerebellar artery (PICA) to PICA bypass, occipital artery (OA) to posterior cerebral artery (PCA) bypass, OA to superior cerebellar artery (SCA) bypass, STA-SCA bypass, and PICA to anterior inferior cerebellar artery bypass. Kawashima et al[11] described a low-flow bypass as one used to cover a relatively small area of vascular irrigation, whereas they described a high-flow bypass as one used for a larger area, such as the entire carotid territory. They also defined a pedicle graft as low flow and defined free interposition grafts (saphenous vein graft or radial artery graft) as high flow.[11]

A high-flow bypass allows a blood flow rate of between 100 and 200 mL/min. A high-flow bypass is used to replace the blood flow when a normal high-flow vessel must be sacrificed.

The term "intermediate flow" is used to describe bypasses with flow rates of approximately 60 to 100 mL/min, which is higher than that provided by a standard pedicled STA-MCA bypass but lower than that provided by a bypass using a saphenous vein graft. Usually intermediate flow is provided by bypasses from the maxillary artery or from the external carotid artery (ECA).[8,12]

Anastomosing Arterial Basins

Bypasses can be characterized on the basis of the anastomosing arterial basins as EC-IC bypasses, intracranial-intracranial (IC-IC) bypasses, or in situ reconstructive procedures and extracranial-extracranial (EC-EC) bypasses (▶ Fig. 10.3). EC-EC procedures in neurosurgical practice involve various reconstructive procedures performed on the carotid and vertebral arteries. In situ intracranial reconstruction techniques are a relatively recent innovation in neurosurgery and were developed after EC-IC anastomoses. IC-IC bypasses are technically more demanding than other bypasses because they require manipulations in a deep operative field.

IC-IC bypasses are most often used in aneurysm surgery (▶ Fig. 10.4). Arterial aneurysms can be excised from the parent vessel with a consequent restoration of vessel integrity by

different IC-IC bypass techniques that do not require harvesting a separate extracranial donor artery, such as by reimplantation or reanastomosis. The term *reanastomosis* means the creation of an end-to-end anastomosis, whereas *reimplantation* means the creation of an end-to-side anastomosis.

Quiñones-Hinojosa and Lawton[13] analyzed a series of in situ vascular reconstructions, including A3-A3, MCA-MCA, and PICA-PICA anastomoses. The authors concluded that in situ reconstructions are less vulnerable to injury or occlusion.[13] Another technique for restoring collateral blood flow is the creation of a side-to-side anastomosis (▶ Fig. 10.5). It is performed between arteries from different sides of the cerebral circulation that lie close to the midline, such as in PICA-PICA and A3-A3 bypasses,[13,14] or between any arteries that run parallel to one another.[15]

Length of the Graft

Another important bypass characteristic is the length of the vascular graft (▶ Fig. 10.6). Bypasses can be classified on the basis of the length of the graft used: short IC-IC grafts (▶ Fig. 10.7), short EC-IC grafts (▶ Fig. 10.8), standard-length grafts (▶ Fig. 10.9), and long grafts (▶ Fig. 10.10).

Liu and Couldwell[5] stated that short grafts have better patency, and they proposed a cervical ICA to supraclinoid ICA saphenous vein bypass via a submandibular pathway. They performed a proximal end-to-end ICA graft anastomosis maximally distal on the neck and made a shorter graft with a more direct route.[5] In 1987, Sato and Kadoya[16] presented three cases in which a long saphenous vein graft was reconstructed after it had been occluded, and the vessels remained patent at the 4-year follow-up. Generally, by long-graft bypass procedures, surgeons mean either a bonnet bypass or a procedure in which grafts are joined to or are proximal to the carotid bifurcation.[17] A tandem bypass is a long-graft procedure using more than one graft to bypass multiple vascular lesions or to lengthen the graft.[18,19] Short-graft bypasses are those that anastomose arteries from the extracranial surface (STA or OA) to the intracranial vessels using a graft (STA to saphenous vein graft to MCA[18]), intracranial interposition grafts, or relatively shorter skull base bypasses (distal cervical ICA to intracranial ICA[5] or

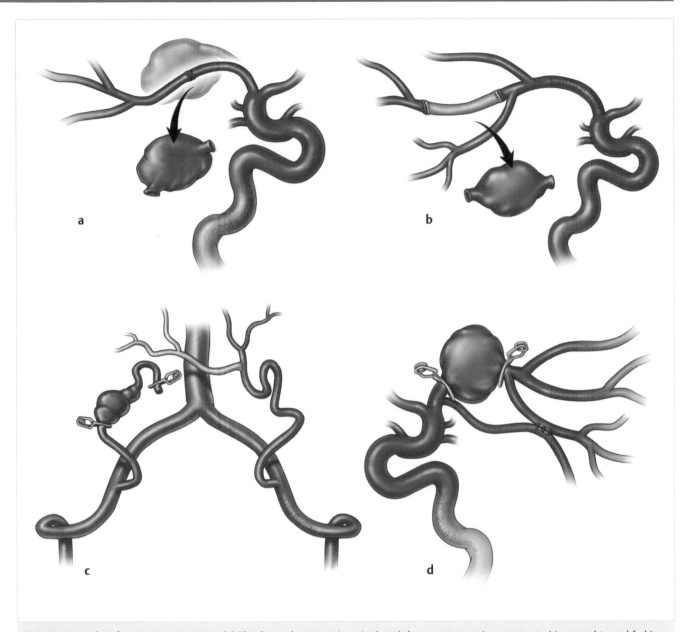

Fig. 10.4 Examples of in situ reconstruction. **(a)** The diseased segment is excised, and the parent artery is reconstructed in an end-to-end fashion (excision-reanastomosis). **(b)** When the two ends cannot be pulled together after resection of the aneurysm, an interposition graft can be used. **(c)** When a branching vessel is compromised or cannot be preserved, it can be transected and reimplanted proximally or on a neighboring vessel with an end-to-side anastomosis (reimplantation). **(d)** A diseased segment may be trapped by clipping and blood flow restored by side-to-side anastomosis of a vessel proximal to the aneurysm to a vessel distal to the aneurysm.

internal maxillary artery [IMA] to MCA[20]). The current recommendation is to use shorter grafts whenever possible. A number of alternative bypasses with shorter grafts have recently been proposed that aim to increase the long-term patency of the grafts compared with the standard ECA to graft to MCA bypass.

Laterality of Bypass Procedure

Another bypass characteristic is laterality (▶ Fig. 10.11). For direct in situ bypasses, the donor artery is usually located on the same side as the recipient artery (▶ Fig. 10.12a). However,

when no suitable donor artery is available on the ipsilateral side, other options are possible, including a bonnet bypass in which blood flow is shunted from the donor artery to the contralateral side (▶ Fig. 10.12b), a tandem bypass, or a long-graft bypass.[21,22] A bilateral bypass may also be used. The term "bilateral" can refer to several variants of bypass. For example, a bilateral bypass can supply blood flow to both anterior cerebral arteries (ACAs) using a Y-shaped or double-barrel graft (▶ Fig. 10.12c).[23] A bilateral bypass can also be performed to revascularize bilateral MCA territories with donor arteries from both sides, usually STA-MCA bypasses in cases of moyamoya disease (▶ Fig. 10.12d).[24]

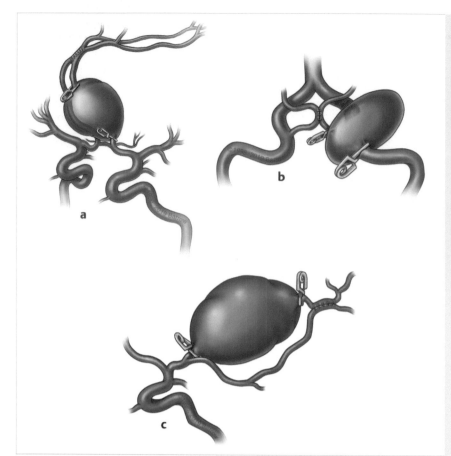

Fig. 10.5 In situ reconstructions using side-to-side anastomosis of neighboring vessels. (a) Anterior cerebral artery (ACA) to ACA anastomosis to provide distal blood flow after the proximal portion of the vessel harboring the aneurysm is sacrificed. (b) Posterior inferior cerebellar artery (PICA) to PICA anastomosis for bypassing a lesion on the proximal portion of one of the PICAs. (c) Middle cerebral artery (MCA) to MCA anastomosis between the anterior temporal artery and a secondary branch of the MCA.

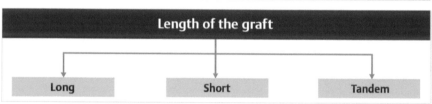

Fig. 10.6 Classification of bypasses on the basis of the length of the vascular graft.

Site of Distal Anastomosis

The spectrum of common sites for distal anastomosis is shown in ▶ Fig. 10.13. Intracranial anastomosis should support blood flow in the distal branches of the sacrificed vessel. The recipient vessel, which is examined preoperatively, should be of appropriate diameter. The diameter of the M1 segment of the MCA is usually 2.4 to 4.6 mm, the diameter of the M2 segment is 1.8 to 3.0 mm, and the diameter of the M4 segment is 0.8 to 1.6 mm.[25] To prevent ischemia during transient occlusion, the recipient vessel should not have a significant number of perforators (most M1 segments have perforators[25]). When the supraclinoid ICA is determined as the recipient vessel, the flow in its distal branches should be supported, which requires a consistent communicant vessel distal to the site of occlusion—either the anterior communicating artery or posterior communicating artery. Revascularization of the posterior circulation deserves special attention, but the bypass strategy and anastomosis principles are the same. The most commonly used recipient vessels are the horizontal segment of the vertebral artery (VA), P2 segment of the PCA, SCA, or PICA.[10]

Site of Proximal Anastomosis

The spectrum of common sites for proximal anastomosis or donor arteries is shown in ▶ Fig. 10.14. In the region of the carotid bifurcation, the common carotid artery, ECA, or ICA can be used as donor vessels. The advantage of an end-to-end anastomosis to the ECA is that the ICA is not occluded during anastomosis, whereas ECA occlusion is well-tolerated. Potential disadvantages include the inability to preserve the STA for bypass. A potential advantage when using the cervical ECA for end-to-side anastomosis is STA preservation without transient ICA occlusion, whereas the blood flow through the ICA is transiently discontinued during the creation of an end-to-side anastomosis on the ICA or common carotid artery.

The subclavian artery can be used as a donor if the carotid arteries are inappropriate. When the subclavian artery is used, the long graft length should be taken into account.[16,26]

Other sources of arterial blood flow are the IMA,[20] petrous ICA,[7] stumps of the STA and OA,[4,27] middle meningeal artery (MMA),[28] posterior auricular artery[29] and different segments of the VA for bypass in the posterior fossa.[14] Several technical difficulties are associated with performing petrous ICA bypasses: exposing the petrous carotid artery is challenging, the greater petrosal nerve usually needs to be sacrificed, the anastomosis is technically difficult, the ICA blood flow is stopped for at least 30 minutes to 1 hour, and the ICA is occluded before the shunt patency is confirmed.[6] The recently described IMA bypass necessitates extensive skull base resection, including removal of the zygoma and temporalis muscle or middle fossa floor.[20,30,31]

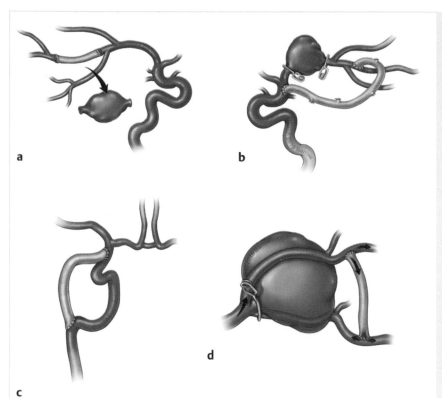

Fig. 10.7 Bypass with short intracranial (IC) to IC interposition graft: **(a)** middle cerebral artery (MCA) to graft to MCA. Bypasses with short IC to IC go-round or "jump" graft: **(b)** supraclinoid internal carotid artery (ICA) to graft to MCA, **(c)** petrous ICA to graft to MCA, and **(d)** MCA to graft to MCA.

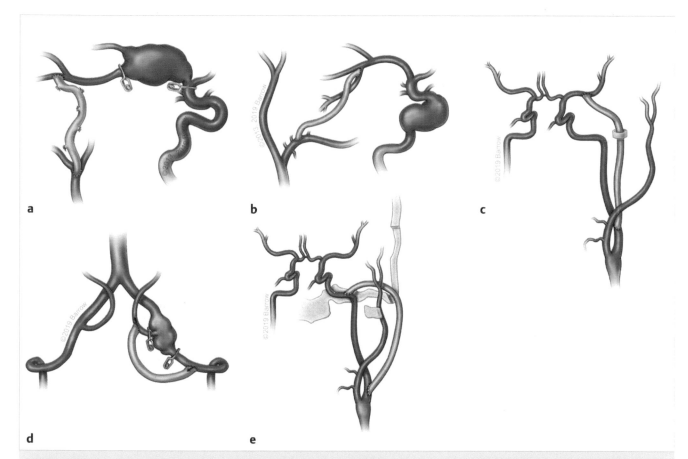

Fig. 10.8 Bypasses with short extracranial to intracranial graft: **(a)** stump superficial temporal artery to graft to middle cerebral artery (MCA), **(b)** internal maxillary artery to graft to MCA, **(c)** distal cervical internal carotid artery (ICA) to graft to MCA, **(d)** vertebral artery to graft to posterior inferior cerebellar artery, and **(e)** external carotid artery/ICA/common carotid artery to graft to petrous ICA.

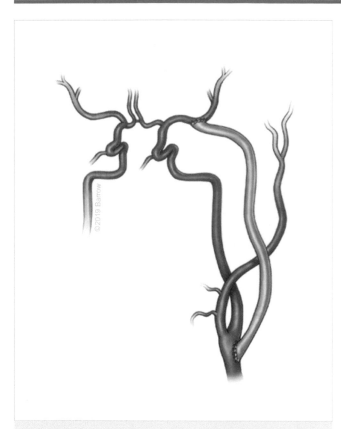

Fig. 10.9 Bypass with standard-length graft: external carotid artery/internal carotid artery/common carotid artery to graft to middle cerebral artery.

This bypass has the potential for injury to the temporomandibular joint, although less traumatic variations have been described.[32]

Options of Distal Anastomosis

A single distal anastomosis is the simplest and most frequently used option; however, complex reconstructions may be necessary (▶ Fig. 10.15). The term *double bypass*, or *double-barrel bypass*, is used to describe different techniques. For example, the term is applied to the bypass procedure when both the frontal and parietal branches of STA are anastomosed with the M4 branches of MCA or the PCA and SCA.[33,34] Another example includes the use of a Y-shaped graft with two distal barrels. This graft can be obtained by harvesting the thoracodorsal axis artery[23] or by modifying a radial artery graft.[35] The term *combined* is usually used for vascular anastomosis combined with indirect revascularization; this type of anastomosis is often used to treat moyamoya disease[24] or is used in combination with an endovascular procedure.[36] A *supportive* bypass is used for blood flow support to the distal branches during the temporary clipping of a proximal part of the vessel for the time needed to create a larger proximal anastomosis. *Sequential* bypass is a type of double bypass in which the recipient vessels are anastomosed to the side and to the end of the donor vessel. This procedure is predominantly used for myocardial revascularization[37] and is an option for intracranial reconstructions. Another technique known as a double reimplantation is a type of sequential bypass in which several efferent recipient branches are implanted at multiple sites into the large caliber proximal vessel or donor graft.[38]

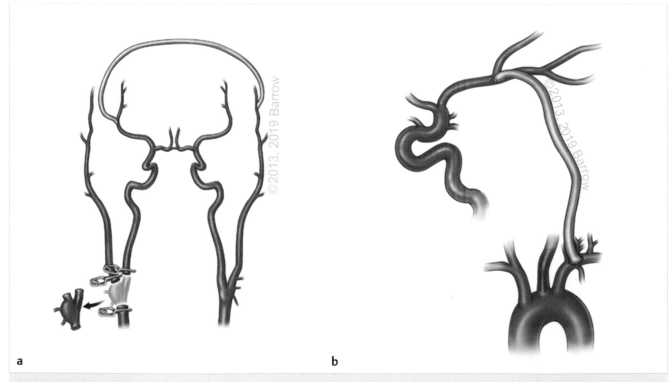

a   b

Fig. 10.10 Bypasses with long grafts: **(a)** superficial temporal artery to graft to middle cerebral artery (MCA) bonnet and **(b)** subclavian artery to graft to MCA.

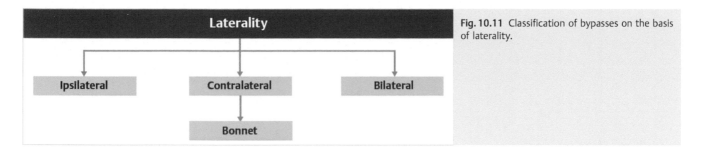

Fig. 10.11 Classification of bypasses on the basis of laterality.

Graft Origin

Grafts can be reasonably classified as pedicled arteries, such as STA grafts and OA grafts, and free vessel grafts, such as radial artery grafts and saphenous vein grafts (▶ Fig. 10.16).[11] The reasons for choosing between radial artery graft and saphenous vein graft are disputable. Saphenous vein graft harvesting usually allows one to obtain a graft that is approximately 25 cm long, whereas radial artery graft harvesting (▶ Fig. 10.17) requires a prolonged dissection, is more invasive, and usually allows one to obtain a graft that is approximately 20 cm long and 2 to 3 mm across.[10]

Grafts are very delicate structures. The possible causes of failure of a saphenous vein graft include endothelial damage caused by venous spasm, overdistension, or direct trauma to the vessel wall during operative manipulation. Applying sutures too tightly to the branch base can cause stenosis at the branching points. Exposing the subendothelial layers to the arterial flow causes inadequate coaptation of the anastomosis. There are other causes of graft failure, such as adventitial tags carelessly left in the vessel lumen, too-vigorous removal of the adventitia, osseous extrinsic compression, and vessel twisting or kinking. Veins also contain valves and should be properly oriented. Saphenous vein grafts are considered to have larger diameter and higher blood flow than radial artery grafts. Radial artery grafts are also susceptible to early vasospasm and intimal hyperplasia. However, applying the pressure distension technique solves the problem of early vasospasm, and calcium channel blockers help in the treatment of intimal hyperplasia of radial artery grafts.[39] The data from the Coronary Artery Surgery Study showed that the long-term patency rate of saphenous vein grafts decreased to 60% after 11 years, and that of radial artery grafts decreased to 91.9% in 5 years.[40] Radial artery grafts seem to have a higher long-term patency and diameter closer to the intracranial arteries than saphenous vein grafts; therefore, they are preferred by many surgeons. A saphenous vein graft is used when the radial artery is not available, is small in diameter (e.g., in children), or when cosmetic considerations must be taken into account (e.g., to avoid dissection on the arm). Other choices for a free graft include a thoracic axis arterial graft,[23] a lingual artery graft,[41] or a portion of STA used as a short vascular graft.[42,43] Synthetic vascular grafts are widely used for large vessels, including the ICA, but they are not suitable for replacing vessels with a smaller diameter. A promising option for patients with no suitable autologous arteries or veins available for grafting is the development of tissue-engineered vascular grafts.[44,45]

Graft Pathway

For a bypass connecting a carotid artery in the neck and one of the intracranial arteries, a vascular graft is usually tunneled either suprazygomatically or subzygomatically (▶ Fig. 10.18). Submandibular graft placement requires removal of the zygomatic arch with muscle retraction and creation of a trough in the middle fossa floor. This route of graft placement provides additional protection compared with a subcutaneous tunnel, and it provides good long-term patency.[5,46] Short EC-IC bypasses from the IMA, distal cervical ICA, or petrous ICA require specific skull-base approaches. A common rule for any approach is that grafts should be aligned in a way to prevent kinking; sometimes a longer loop-graft trajectory is better than a short graft with a change of flow direction at a sharp angle.[42,47]

10.2.2 General Principles of Indirect Neurosurgical Bypass Procedures

In some clinical situations, indirect bypasses are the only available method of benefit for the patient, and in some cases they can be used in combination with direct anastomoses.[48,49,50,51]

Depending on the type of tissue that is surgically attached to the brain surface, indirect anastomoses can be divided into the following types:
1. Encephalomyosynangiosis (EMS) (▶ Fig. 10.19a)
2. Encephaloduroarteriosynangiosis (EDAS) (▶ Fig. 10.19b, c)
3. A combination of EMS and EDAS (▶ Fig. 10.19d)
4. Encephalomyoarteriosynangiosis (EMAS)
5. Encephalogaleosynangiosis (EGS)
6. Omentum transplantation
7. Turnover of dural arteries

Studies have shown significant increase of blood flow after multiple cranial bur holes with dura incisions were placed in the temporal region (▶ Fig. 10.19e).[52,53]

EMS involves the inner part of the temporalis muscle, separated into two fragments and placed over the cortex. After this operation, the deep branches of the temporalis artery develop anastomoses to the cortical branches of the MCA.

EDAS or onlay bypass[54] is used when direct anastomosis of the STA and the cortical branches of the MCA cannot be performed. The STA branches are placed on the surface of the brain and fixed to the dura.[55,56]

In special cases, EGS, *omentum transplantation*, and *trephinations* can be performed, but these procedures have limited utility.[52,53]

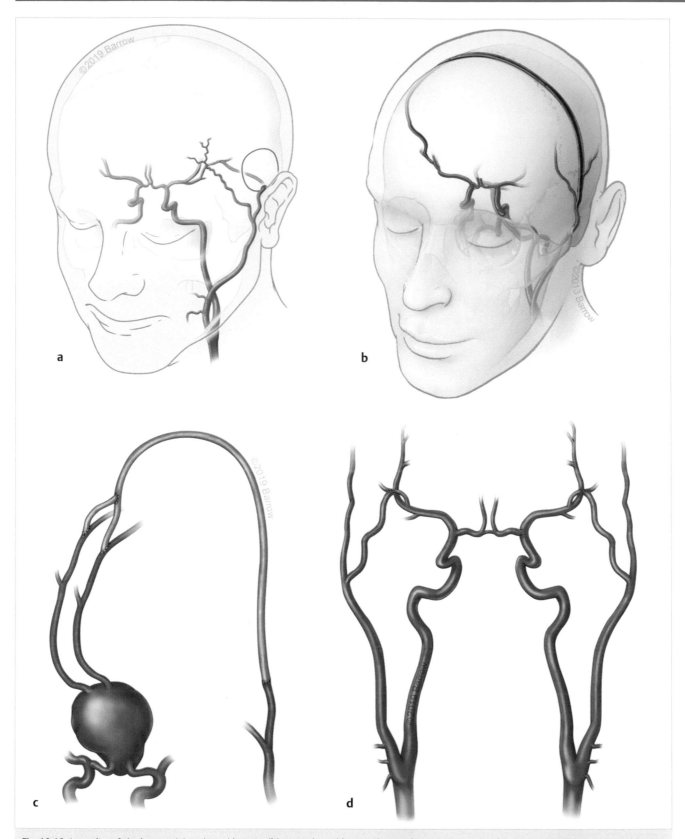

Fig. 10.12 Laterality of the bypass. **(a)** Ipsilateral bypass. **(b)** Contralateral bypass (bonnet bypass as an example). **(c)** Double-barrel, Y-shaped bypass tailored from the radial artery to cover the territories of both anterior cerebral arteries, and **(d)** bilateral superficial temporal artery to middle cerebral artery bypasses for the territories of both middle cerebral arteries.

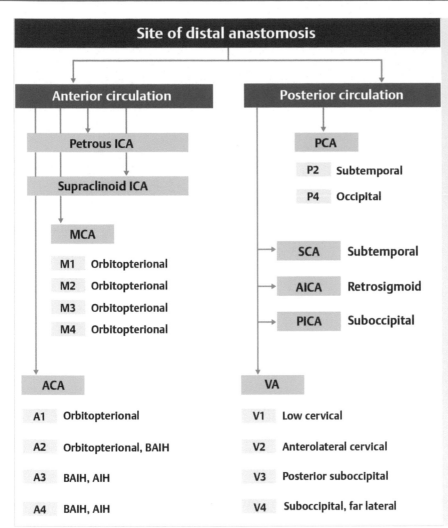

Fig. 10.13 Classification of bypasses on the basis of the site of distal anastomosis (with recipient vessel). Abbreviations: A1–A4, segments of anterior cerebral artery; ACA, anterior cerebral artery; AIH, anterior interhemispheric; BAIH, basal anterior interhemispheric; ICA, internal carotid artery; M1–M4, segments of middle cerebral artery; MCA, middle cerebral artery; P2, P4, branches of the posterior cerebral artery; PCA, posterior cerebral artery; PICA, posterior inferior cerebellar artery; SCA, superior cerebellar artery; V1–V4, segments of vertebral artery; VA, vertebral artery.

The results of EDAS, EMS, and EGS, and other indirect bypasses have been demonstrated in a number of studies.[57,58,59] These types of synangiosis procedures are still widely used for the treatment of moyamoya disease, especially in children.[60] The small vessel diameters in patients with moyamoya make anastomosis difficult to perform, so indirect bypass is often the only surgical option for these patients. Several studies have shown that a period of 3 to 12 months is needed for the development of new blood vasculature in the brain after indirect bypass is performed.[50,61]

While controversy of selection of direct versus indirect bypass for adult moyamoya patients in ongoing,[62] it is thought that, with established proficiency in microsurgical technique, direct bypasses are generally more effective in terms of immediate angiographically evident revascularization[63,64] and restoration of cerebrovascular reserve capacity. EDAS was minimally effective in an older cohort of patients.[48,49,50]

Combined revascularization techniques (direct plus indirect bypasses) are generally preferred in patients with moyamoya, because these techniques combine the benefits of immediate flow augmentation through direct bypass and the creation of maximally favorable conditions for further neovascularization.

10.3 Operative Techniques for Direct Bypass Procedures

10.3.1 Bypasses for Blood Flow Augmentation

A single or double low-flow bypass can be performed using branches of the STA. Double low-flow anastomosis, frontal STA-graft-ACA, and temporal STA-MCA may be used for the revascularization of both ACA and MCA territories. Usually, suprasylvian and infrasylvian branches of the MCA are used for the recipient vessel. The double STA-MCA bypass is applicable when the MCA bifurcation is occluded or when cerebral blood flow in both the frontal and the temporal lobes is impaired.[49,65] This bypass is appropriate for the trapping of complicated MCA aneurysms. Double bypass also offers an opportunity for neurosurgeons to develop their technical skills, as one of the anastomoses can be performed by a less-experienced neurosurgeon under the guidance of the main neurosurgeon.

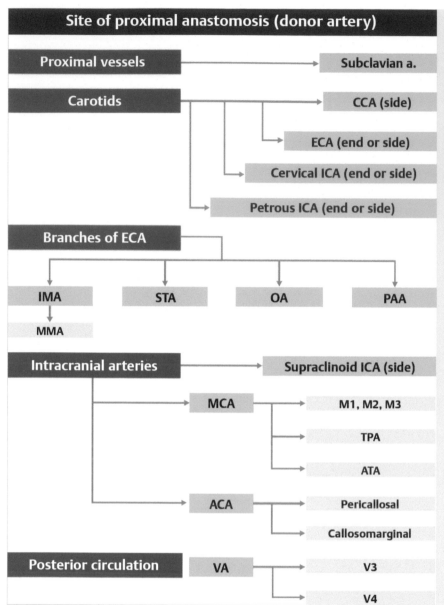

Fig. 10.14 Classification of bypasses on the basis of the site of proximal anastomosis (with donor vessel). Abbreviations: a., artery; ACA, anterior cerebral artery; ATA, anterior temporal artery; CCA, common carotid artery; ECA, external carotid artery; ICA, internal carotid artery; IMA, internal maxillary artery; M1–M3, segments of middle cerebral artery; MCA, middle cerebral artery; MMA, middle meningeal artery; OA, occipital artery; PAA, posterior auricular artery; STA, superficial temporal artery; TPA, temporopolar artery; V3, V4, segments of vertebral artery; VA, vertebral artery.

STA-MCA Bypass

The basic techniques of low-flow bypass surgery can be demonstrated by the example of STA-MCA anastomosis, which is one of the standard bypass procedures for brain revascularization.[66]

Preoperative Planning

During preoperative planning, appropriate donor and recipient vessels are chosen by reviewing conventional angiography images, computed tomography (CT) angiography images, or magnetic resonance angiography (MRA) images of the ECA and ICA.

Patient Positioning

The patient is placed in the supine position with the head fixed in a frame and turned to the contralateral side, and the ipsilateral shoulder is raised with a cushion. The head should be flat to tilted down to facilitate drainage from the operative field.

Electrophysiology neuromonitoring probes are attached to the patient's head. STA branches are marked on the skin with indelible marker under mini-Doppler navigation (▶ Fig. 10.20). Then, the hair is shaved to a width of 1 to 2 cm along the planned incision line. The skin is prepared using standard aseptic protocol without skin infiltration or local anesthesia, which can cause vessel spasm or injury.

Skin Incision and Craniotomy

The type of skin incision used for bypass procedures varies between clinics and surgeons and according to the needs of the patient (▶ Fig. 10.21). General considerations for the skin incision are STA course, hairline, and adequate approach to the recipient artery (the MCA). In general, an incision that follows the STA is most commonly used.

One of two types of craniotomy is usually used: a regular frontotemporal craniotomy or a small "keyhole" craniotomy. A

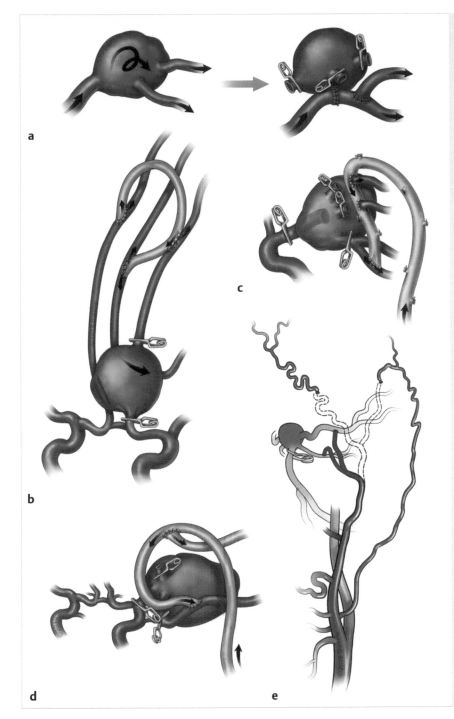

Fig. 10.15 Variants of complex reconstructions. **(a)** Combination of M1-M2 end-to-end reanastomosis and M2-M2 end-to-side reimplantation. **(b)** In situ jump graft sequential bypass: end-to-side radial artery graft to pericallosal artery (PcaA), side-to-side radial artery graft to PcaA, and end-to-side radial artery graft to callosomarginal artery anastomoses. **(c)** Extracranial-intracranial (EC-IC) sequential bypass with double reimplantations: external carotid artery (ECA) to saphenous vein graft to M2 (side-to-end), ECA to saphenous vein graft to M2 (side-to-end), and ECA to saphenous vein graft to M3 (end-to-side). **(d)** EC-IC sequential bypass with reimplantation: ECA to graft to M2 (side-to-end) and ECA to graft to M2 (end-to-side). **(e)** Double-barrel superficial temporal artery (STA) to superior cerebellar artery and STA to posterior cerebral artery bypass.

targeted keyhole bypass can be performed through a small craniotomy using navigation. In this approach, the keyhole position is planned according to the recipient artery position and chosen preoperatively using brain metabolic, perfusion, and angiographic data obtained from MRA, positron emission tomography, and CT.[65] The craniotomy should be large enough to allow selection between a number of surface vessels, as the imaging and exposed appearance do not always correspond perfectly.

A linear incision can be used for a single bypass through a small craniotomy. A J-shaped incision is usually used for a double bypass. A single incision can be used for the temporal STA

branch, with a small supportive incision placed for additional dissection of the frontal STA branch for a double bypass through a small craniotomy as described by Yoshimura et al.[67] A J-shaped incision is created as follows: the first, ascending part of the incision is performed in the projection of the temporal branch of the STA. After the STA is dissected, the incision is prolonged anteriorly, and a craniotomy is performed above the site where the MCA emerges from the sylvian fissure. The frontal branch of the STA can then be easily dissected from the inside of the scalp flap. A craniotomy with a 4 cm diameter is usually adequate for exposing the appropriate recipient artery. The center of the craniotomy is located on a line perpendicular to the

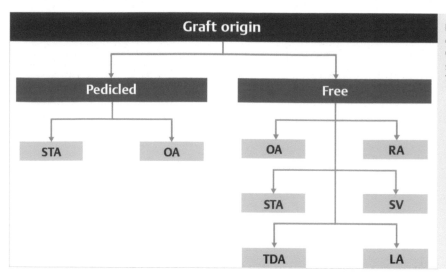

Fig. 10.16 Classification of bypasses on the basis of graft origin. Abbreviations: LA, lingual artery; OA, occipital artery; RA, radial artery; STA, superficial temporal artery; SV, saphenous vein; TDA, thoracodorsal axis artery.

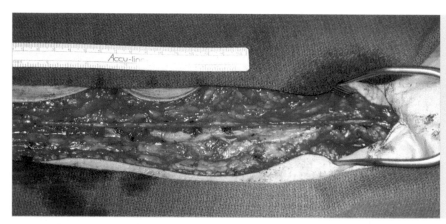

Fig. 10.17 Intraoperative photograph of dissection of the radial artery for use as a graft. (Reproduced with permission from Spetzler RF, Koos WT: Color Atlas of Microneurosurgery 2e. Vol. 3 Intra- and Extracranial Revascularization and Intraspinal Pathology, New York: Thieme, 2000.)

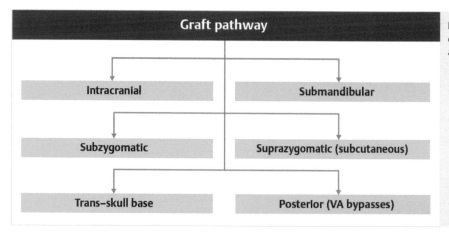

Fig. 10.18 Classification of bypasses on the basis of graft pathway. Abbreviation: VA, vertebral artery.

orbitoauricular line, 6 cm above the external auditory meatus. This procedure consistently exposes the vessels around the angular gyrus (▶ Fig. 10.21a).[68]

Meticulous hemostasis throughout the operation is necessary to prevent obstruction of the view by blood and cerebrospinal fluid during microsurgery suturing, to prevent postoperative hematomas, and to preserve hemoglobin with a hematocrit at 30 to 35% so that brain ischemia is avoided, especially in pediatric patients with low total blood volume.[69]

Dissection of the STA

To begin the dissection, the sides of the incision are retracted with fishhooks. High-powered bipolar microforceps (Codman: 60–70; Codman & Shurtleff, Inc.) with suction are used to dissect the STA. When it is free at both ends, the temporalis muscle is incised, and the craniotomy is performed. Once a surface recipient vessel is identified, a temporary clip is applied to the proximal end of the STA, and the distal end is ligated and

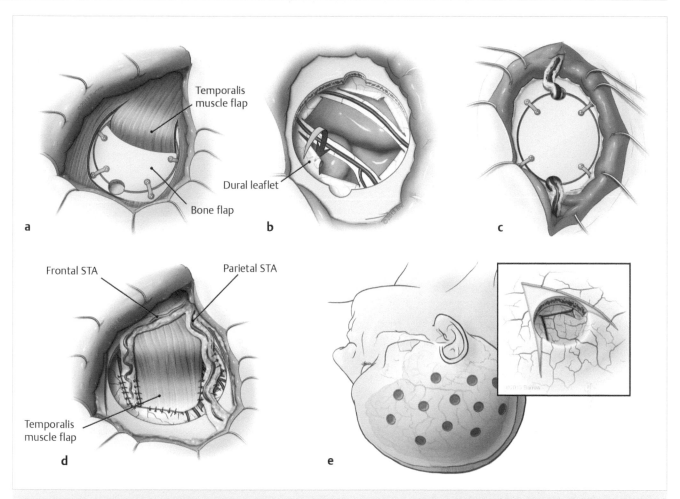

Temporalis
muscle flap

Dural leaflet

Bone flap

a

b

c

Frontal STA

Parietal STA

Temporalis
muscle flap

d

e

Fig. 10.19 Various indirect bypasses. **(a)** Encephalomyosynangiosis (EMS) involves placement of the inner layer of the temporalis muscle over the brain surface. **(b)** Encephaloduroarteriosynangiosis (EDAS) involves leaflets of dura inverted under the skull while the middle meningeal artery is left intact and **(c)** relocation of the dissected superficial temporal artery over the brain surface. **(d)** Combination of EMS and EDAS. **(e)** Multiple trephinations with dural incisions and placement of the fascial leaflets under the dura.

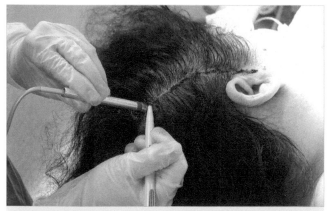

Fig. 10.20 Superficial temporal artery is marked on the skin with surgical marker under Doppler navigation for planning the location of the incision.

cut. The dissected portion of the vessel is washed with heparinized normal saline, moistened with papaverine, and kept with care.

After the STA is dissected from the inner side of the scalp, the galea should be carefully repaired using absorbable sutures to preserve blood flow to the scalp.

Preparation of Bloodless Operative Field

The dura mater is fixed to the bone edge and opened in an X-shaped fashion, oriented to the site of the donor vessel entrance. The MMA can provide collateral blood flow through the dura mater to the brain surface, so it should be preserved if possible. To preserve the MMA, it may be helpful to perform a modified craniotomy with a protective bony ridge over the MMA that is subsequently removed with a ball drill as described by Kuroda and Houkin.[24]

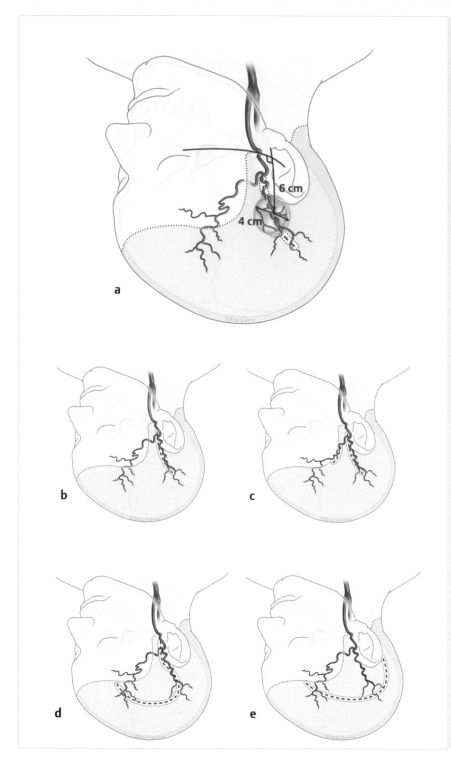

Fig. 10.21 Variety of skin incisions for superficial temporal artery (STA) to middle cerebral artery bypass surgery. Planned skin incisions are represented by the *blue dashed lines*. **(a)** Mapping the craniotomy site.[68] The center of the craniotomy is located 6 cm above the external acoustic meatus, on the line, perpendicular to the orbitomeatal line. The craniotomy is usually 4 cm in diameter. **(b)** Single linear incision. **(c)** Two linear incisions for dissection of both STA branches. **(d)** J-shaped incision. **(e)** U-shaped incision.

Appropriate M4 branches are visualized and prepared by sharp subarachnoid dissection. Small branches on the back wall of the artery are then cauterized with low heat and divided. The segment of prepared recipient artery should be at least three times as long as the diameter of the STA.[70] In most cases, for double bypass, two recipient vessels should be exposed, the suprasylvian and infrasylvian M4 branches. Colored silicone rubber should be placed under the recipient artery to clearly visualize the almost-transparent walls of the recipient vessel.

Small sheets of cotton pads are used to separate the operative field with a continuous suction drainage left under them. This drainage helps to eliminate fluid and blood from the operative field and facilitates good operative conditions.

Anastomosis Creation

For proper creation of anastomoses, trainees should obtain the skills of meticulous microsurgery suturing through continuous

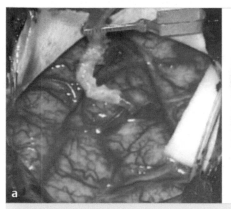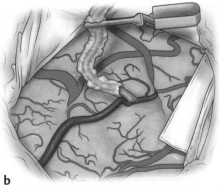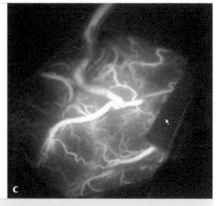

Fig. 10.22 (a) Intraoperative photograph and (b) illustration of operative field after superficial temporal artery to middle cerebral artery bypass. (c) Confirmation of patency after clip removal using indocyanine green videoangiography. (Figs. 10.22a,c are provided courtesy of Dr. Ken-ichiro Kikuta, MD.)

laboratory training. The end of the STA donor artery is released from its surrounding adventitia, and the lumen is widened in a fish–mouth-like shape. Clear visualization of the donor and recipient orifices is essential. For this purpose, staining with pyoctanin blue (also known as gentian violet, available as surgical skin marker) or methylene blue dye is very helpful.

After two temporary clips (usually arteriovenous malformation clips, but microaneurysm clips may be substituted) are applied to the recipient artery, the arteriotomy is carried out and adjustments of the anastomotic sites are performed. Tenting suture can be helpful for arteriotomy in large recipient arteries. Tenting the suture facilitates accurate cutting with the scissors. If the diameter of the anastomosis is small (< 1 mm), a linear arteriotomy can be performed with the needle tip of an insulin syringe. The arterial lumen and surroundings are irrigated with a heparinized saline solution. After completion of the anastomosis, minor blood leakage can be repaired by using Surgicel (Ethicon US, LLC) or a piece of muscle.

Confirmation of Patency

Patency of the anastomosis is verified by intraoperative video-angiography using indocyanine green or fluorescein sodium[71] (▶ Fig. 10.22). Blood flow in the donor vessel is also verified by nonquantitative or quantitative Doppler ultrasonography during the wound closure. Although intraoperative digital subtraction angiography has been the gold standard for the evaluation of graft patency, it has its own limitations, such as high cost, invasiveness, and ionizing radiation.

Wound Closure

A small opening is incised in the dura and muscle for the donor artery entrance. The dura mater is tightly sutured and secured with fibrin glue. The bone flap with a slot for donor artery entrance is fixed with titanium plates with special care given to avoid bending, compression, or traumatization to the donor vessels. The postoperative wound is sutured in layers with separate stitches for the aponeurosis, and skin clips stabilize tension of the scalp flap to prevent ischemia, necrosis, and leakage of cerebrospinal fluid and to decrease the risk of infection.

STA-ACA Bypass

Direct STA-ACA anastomosis is essential in rare cases with pronounced ischemia in the ACA territory. The whole procedure is performed in the same fashion as the STA-MCA bypass, but with some distinct characteristics.

The dissection of the frontal branch of the STA should be as long as possible to enable easy and safe handling. The recipient vessel is the cortical ACA branch close to the midline. The frontal branch of the STA and the ACA are smaller in diameter than either the temporal STA branch or the MCA. This size difference may render the bypass more challenging. In rare cases in which the frontal branch of the STA runs extremely caudally and close to the temporal branch of the facial nerve, only the distal portion of the frontal STA branch should be dissected from the scalp to avoid postoperative frontal muscle palsy.[1]

A saphenous vein graft, radial artery graft, or the contralateral STA can be used as an interposition graft to elongate the donor vessel for an STA-graft-A3-A4 bypass. This procedure requires additional end-to-end anastomosis of the STA to an interposition graft. This approach was successful as a supportive bypass for the treatment of a recurrent anterior communicating artery aneurysm after coil embolization followed by trapping.[39]

STA-PCA or OA-PCA Bypass

The STA-PCA or OA-PCA bypasses are used for brain ischemia in the PCA area in moyamoya disease and as a support for the treatment of complex PCA aneurysms.[33] Patients with moyamoya who have PCA lesions are considered to have a higher risk for subsequent ischemic stroke because the PCA often acts as a collateral blood flow reserve to ICA territory. Revascularization for both the PCA and MCA areas should be planned in such cases.[24,72]

It is possible to revascularize the PCA territory by indirect bypass procedures performed over the occipital lobe, by direct anastomoses to the P2 segment of PCA through the subtemporal approach to the ambient and crural cisterns,[73] or to the more distal PCA branches through the occipital interhemispheric approach.[74,75] OA is usually the preferred donor vessel, but STA may also be chosen if available in sufficient length. Anastomoses to the PCA are significantly more complex than bypasses in the MCA circulation due to the narrowness of the operative approaches and the abundance of critical brainstem perforating vessels. For distal PCA aneurysms, bypasses are reserved for patients who cannot undergo primary stenting with coiling or clip wrapping.[76,77]

OA as a Donor Vessel

Revascularization of the posterior cranial fossa can be performed using the OA or STA, or by using grafts to borrow arterial flow from the VA. The OA is very tortuous and lies deeper than the STA.[78] After exiting the occipital groove, the OA runs superomedially in the posterior triangle through the longissimus capitis and semispinalis capitis muscles and usually pierces the trapezius attachment to the superior nuchal line, although sometimes it exists between the trapezius and semispinalis capitis to continue to run superiorly in the superficial fascia. The length of the OA is usually sufficient for a posterior fossa bypass but is not always sufficient for MCA anastomosis.

10.3.2 Bypass for Blood Flow Replacement

The creation of bypasses for blood flow replacement is a technically demanding procedure. It is an artistic procedure with many nuances that differ across neurosurgical centers. Martin has described the surgical techniques for EC-IC bypass in detail for the treatment of aneurysms.[79] Flow demand should be estimated before planning surgery so that an adequate donor vessel can be chosen. Usually, an interposition graft from the carotid artery is preferred because it is a high-flow bypass; however, a double-STA bypass[80] or a shorter bypass from the maxillary artery could be considered. In this chapter, we have presented the main operative technical steps for performing an EC-IC high-flow bypass from the carotid bifurcation using an interposition graft.

Carotid Artery to Interposition Graft to MCA Bypass

Preoperative Planning

For a carotid artery to interposition graft to MCA bypass, appropriate recipient vessels are selected using ICA injection digital subtraction angiography and MRA or CT angiography.[81] During the angiography, if occlusion is planned, the balloon occlusion test may be performed to assess the tolerance of the parent vessel to occlusion. The donor vessel is assessed using MRA of the neck or common carotid injection digital subtraction angiography. The rationale for choosing a radial artery graft or a saphenous vein graft is described above. For radial artery graft harvesting, the Allen test should be performed before the operation to confirm the patency of the ulnar artery. This test is routinely used by anesthesiologists before arterial catheter placement. For the harvesting part of the procedure, the potential graft and its branches must be marked on the skin with indelible marker under Doppler navigation; the cervical and cranial approaches should also be marked.

Graft Harvesting

The patient is placed in a supine position with the head fixed in a Mayfield or Sugita head holder. The neck is slightly extended (10 degrees) and elevated to increase venous drainage. The head is then rotated 75 degrees away from the side of approach. Both legs are prepared from the ankles to the thighs for saphenous vein harvesting, or an arm is prepared for radial artery harvesting. The harvesting procedure can be performed by cardiac or peripheral vascular surgeons[51] or by a second team of neurosurgeons. Endoscopic harvesting (VasoView, Maquet Holding B.V. & Co. KG, Rastatt, Germany) is a minimally invasive alternative to the traditional open long-incision procedure.[82]

Neck Dissection

The neck is prepared the same way as it is for an endarterectomy ipsilaterally to the craniotomy. The carotid bifurcation and the ECA should be dissected free enough to allow ECA clips to be applied distally and proximally, allowing the bifurcation and the ECA to be mobilized.

Craniotomy

Because a high-flow bypass is usually used for the reconstruction of deeply located proximal cerebral arteries (e.g., the ICA, the M1 and M2 segments of the MCA, and the A2 segment of the ACA), the selection of the craniotomy site depends on the primary pathologic entity. Usually a pterional craniotomy or an orbitozygomatic approach with wide Sylvian fissure dissection is used to expose the proximal intracranial recipient vessel.[70] Some surgeons also perform an additional zygomatic osteotomy and drill a groove on the bone according to the graft course to increase the space available for the graft.

Tunneling of the Graft

Subcutaneous dissections with Kelly clamps between the craniotomy and the cervical incision are used to create the tunnel. The tunnel goes under the zygomatic arch and behind the mandible (▶ Fig. 10.23). A pediatric chest tube is then passed from the cervical incision upward. The graft is placed into the tube and pulled through using a suture. After the first anastomosis is completed, the graft is allowed to bleed so that it straightens and is not rotated in the tunnel. Blue marking on the same side on both ends of the graft is also helpful to indicate when the graft is twisted. Alternatively, the graft can be pulled through an opening made in the middle fossa floor.[46]

Distal Anastomosis

Distal anastomosis is performed first, before the proximal anastomosis, because the free end of the graft allows extra mobility and allows the graft to be flipped for more comfortable suturing of the back wall of the anastomosis. The suturing method is the same as that used for the STA-MCA bypass, but this procedure is more difficult due to the greater depth of the operative field. Because distal anastomosis involves working at such depth, it requires the neurosurgeon to use instruments with longer handles and to have more precise manual skills. Small sheets of cottonoids with a continuous suction drainage left under them are

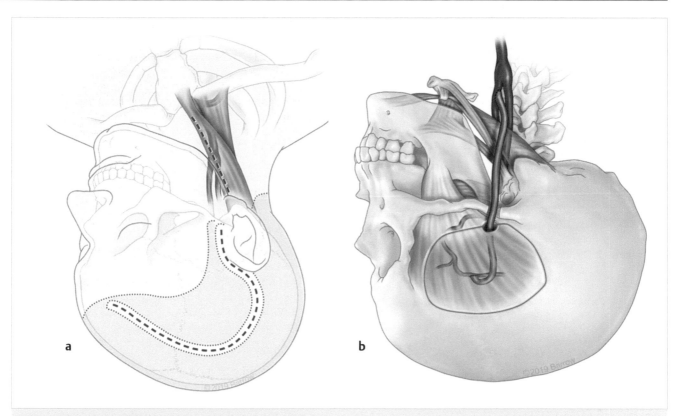

Fig. 10.23 Schematic of external carotid artery to graft to middle cerebral artery high-flow bypass. (a) Skin incision (*blue dashed line*) for carotid approach and frontal-temporal craniotomy. (b) Placement of graft.

used to protect the surrounding brain. This drainage helps eliminate fluid and blood from the operative field and facilitates good operative conditions. A sheet of colored silicone material is placed under the recipient artery to allow the sutured segments to be clearly seen.

Excimer laser-assisted nonocclusive anastomosis is an alternative technology to hand suturing and is associated with a high patency rate.[83]

Proximal Anastomosis

When the STA is not used as a donor vessel, the graft is usually anastomosed to the ECA in an end-to-end fashion. Due to the potential size mismatch, the saphenous vein graft/radial artery graft opening may have to be slightly enlarged by using an oblique cut or fish-mouthing the vessel. Size 7–0 Prolene (Ethicon, USA, LLC) sutures are usually used. End-to-side anastomosis is used for a combined bypass to preserve the ipsilateral STA and MMA. When a vascular graft is used, the temporary clips should be released to allow the recipient and donor vessel to bleed in sequential order to remove air and potential clots before the last suture is tied. In addition, after the last sutures are tied, the ECA clip should be removed before the ICA clip to allow flushing of any possible blood clots and residual air from the graft and anastomosis toward the distal ECA branches rather than toward the ICA.

ICA Ligation

The ICA should be ligated at the bifurcation even with the ECA. Leaving a stump of the ICA can cause thrombosis and can be a potential source of embolism.[20,84]

Confirmation of Patency

Patency is confirmed in the same manner as for a low-flow bypass.

Wound Closure

Wound closure is performed in the same manner as for a low-flow bypass.

References

[1] Yamada S, Brauer FS, Purtzer T, Haywqard W, Hill TW, Hamamura RK. MCA occlusion during STA-MCA anastomosis does not compromise cerebral metabolic or electrical activity. In: Spetzler RF, Carter LP, Selman WR, Martin WA, eds. Cerebral Revascularization for Stroke. New York, NY: Stratton-Thieme; 1985:29–40

[2] Batjer H, Samson D. Use of extracranial-intracranial bypass in the management of symptomatic vasospasm. Neurosurgery; 19(2):235–246

[3] Amin-Hanjani S, Du X, Mlinarevich N, Meglio G, Zhao M, Charbel FT. The cut flow index: an intraoperative predictor of the success of extracranial-intracranial bypass for occlusive cerebrovascular disease. Neurosurgery; 56(1) Suppl:75–85, discussion 75–85

[4] Amin-Hanjani S, Alaraj A, Charbel FT. Flow replacement bypass for aneurysms: decision-making using intraoperative blood flow measurements. Acta Neurochir (Wien); 152(6):1021–1032, discussion 1032

[5] Liu JK, Couldwell WT. Interpositional carotid artery bypass strategies in the surgical management of aneurysms and tumors of the skull base. Neurosurg Focus; 14(3):e2

[6] Ramina R, Meneses MS, Pedrozo AA, Arruda WO, Borges G. Saphenous vein graft bypass in the treatment of giant cavernous sinus aneurysms: report of two cases. Arq Neuropsiquiatr; 58(1):162–168

[7] Spetzler RF, Fukushima T, Martin N, Zabramski JM. Petrous carotid-to-intradural carotid saphenous vein graft for intracavernous giant aneurysm, tumor, and occlusive cerebrovascular disease. J Neurosurg; 73(4):496–501

[8] Wessels L, Hecht N, Vajkoczy P. Bypass in neurosurgery-indications and techniques. Neurosurg Rev(Mar):13

[9] da Silva HB, Messina-Lopez M, Sekhar LN. Bypasses and reconstruction for complex brain aneurysms. Methodist DeBakey Cardiovasc J; 10(4):224–233

[10] Mohit AA, Sekhar LN, Natarajan SK, Britz GW, Ghodke B. High-flow bypass grafts in the management of complex intracranial aneurysms. Neurosurgery; 60(2) Suppl 1:ONS105–ONS122, discussion ONS122–ONS123

[11] Kawashima M, Rhoton AL , Jr, Tanriover N, Ulm AJ, Yasuda A, Fujii K. Microsurgical anatomy of cerebral revascularization. Part I: anterior circulation. J Neurosurg; 102(1):116–131

[12] Yu Z, Shi X, Brohi SR, Qian H, Liu F, Yang Y. Measurement of blood flow in an intracranial artery bypass from the internal maxillary artery by intraoperative duplex sonography. J Ultrasound Med; 36(2):439–447

[13] Quiñones-Hinojosa A, Lawton MT. In situ bypass in the management of complex intracranial aneurysms: technique application in 13 patients. Neurosurgery; 57(1) Suppl:140–145, discussion 140–145

[14] Lemole GM , Jr, Henn J, Javedan S, Deshmukh V, Spetzler RF. Cerebral revascularization performed using posterior inferior cerebellar artery-posterior inferior cerebellar artery bypass. Report of four cases and literature review. J Neurosurg; 97(1):219–223

[15] Bederson JB, Spetzler RF. Anastomosis of the anterior temporal artery to a secondary trunk of the middle cerebral artery for treatment of a giant M1 segment aneurysm. Case report. J Neurosurg; 76(5):863–866

[16] Sato S, Kadoya S. EC-IC bypass surgery using a long vein graft—reconstructive procedures for the occluded long vein grafts [in Japanese]. No Shinkei Geka; 15(8):885–890

[17] Kalani MY, Kalb S, Martirosyan NL, et al. Cerebral revascularization and carotid artery resection at the skull base for treatment of advanced head and neck malignancies. J Neurosurg; 118(3):637–642

[18] Little JR, Furlan AJ, Bryerton B. Short vein grafts for cerebral revascularization. J Neurosurg; 59(3):384–388

[19] Auguste KI, Quiñones-Hinojosa A, Lawton MT. The tandem bypass: subclavian artery-to-middle cerebral artery bypass with dacron and saphenous vein grafts. Technical case report. Surg Neurol; 56(3):164–169

[20] Abdulrauf SI, Sweeney JM, Mohan YS, Palejwala SK. Short segment internal maxillary artery to middle cerebral artery bypass: a novel technique for extracranial-to-intracranial bypass. Neurosurgery; 68(3):804–808, discussion 808–809

[21] Kalani MY, Rangel-Castilla L, Ramey W, et al. Indications and results of direct cerebral revascularization in the modern era. World Neurosurg; 83(3):345–350

[22] Spetzler RF, Roski RA, Rhodes RS, Modic MT. The "bonnet bypass". Case report. J Neurosurg; 53(5):707–709

[23] Jain A, O'Neill K, Patel MC, Kirkpatrick N, Sivathasan N, Nanchahal J. Extracranial-intracranial bypass of the bilateral anterior cerebral circulation using a thoracodorsal axis artery-graft. Asian J Neurosurg; 7(4):203–205

[24] Kuroda S, Houkin K. Bypass surgery for moyamoya disease: concept and essence of sugical techniques. Neurol Med Chir (Tokyo); 52(5):287–294

[25] Yasargil MG. Microneurosurgery: Microsurgical Anatomy of the Basal Cisterns and Vessels of the Brain, Diagnostic Studies, General Operative Techniques and Pathological Considerations of the Intracranial Aneurysms. Vol. 1. Stuttgart: Georg Thieme Verlag; 1984

[26] Spetzler RF, Rhodes RS, Roski RA, Likavec MJ. Subclavian to middle cerebral artery saphenous vein bypass graft. J Neurosurg; 53(4):465–469

[27] Fujimura M, Inoue T, Shimizu H, Tominaga T. Occipital artery-anterior inferior cerebellar artery bypass with microsurgical trapping for exclusively intrameatal anterior inferior cerebellar artery aneurysm manifesting as subarachnoid hemorrhage. Case report. Neurol Med Chir (Tokyo); 52(6):435–438

[28] Miller CF , II, Spetzler RF, Kopaniky DJ. Middle meningeal to middle cerebral arterial bypass for cerebral revascularization. Case report. J Neurosurg; 50(6):802–804

[29] Horiuchi T, Kusano Y, Asanuma M, Hongo K. Posterior auricular artery-middle cerebral artery bypass for additional surgery of moyamoya disease. Acta Neurochir (Wien); 154(3):455–456

[30] Nossek E, Costantino PD, Eisenberg M, et al. Internal maxillary artery-middle cerebral artery bypass: infratemporal approach for subcranial-intracranial (SC-IC) bypass. Neurosurgery; 75(1):87–95

[31] Eller JL, Sasaki-Adams D, Sweeney JM, Abdulrauf SI. Localization of the internal maxillary artery for extracranial-to-intracranial bypass through the middle cranial fossa: a cadaveric study. J Neurol Surg B Skull Base; 73(1):48–53

[32] Yağmurlu K, Kalani MYS, Martirosyan NL, et al. The maxillary artery to middle cerebral artery bypass: a novel technique for exposure of the maxillary artery. World Neurosurg; 100:540–550

[33] Kalani MY, Ramey W, Albuquerque FC, et al. Revascularization and aneurysm surgery: techniques, indications, and outcomes in the endovascular era. Neurosurgery; 74(5):482–497, discussion 497–498

[34] Kalani MY, Hu YC, Spetzler RF. A double-barrel superficial temporal artery-to-superior cerebellar artery (STA-SCA) and STA-to-posterior cerebral artery (STA-PCA) bypass for revascularization of the basilar apex. J Clin Neurosci; 20 (6):887–889

[35] Dengler J, Kato N, Vajkoczy P. The Y-shaped double-barrel bypass in the treatment of large and giant anterior communicating artery aneurysms. J Neurosurg; 118(2):444–450

[36] Hacein-Bey L, Connolly ES , Jr, Mayer SA, Young WL, Pile-Spellman J, Solomon RA. Complex intracranial aneurysms: combined operative and endovascular approaches. Neurosurgery; 43(6):1304–1312, discussion 1312–1313

[37] Kabinejadian F, Chua LP, Ghista DN, Sankaranarayanan M, Tan YS. A novel coronary artery bypass graft design of sequential anastomoses. Ann Biomed Eng; 38(10):3135–3150

[38] Mirzadeh Z, Sanai N, Lawton MT. The azygos anterior cerebral artery bypass: double reimplantation technique for giant anterior communicating artery aneurysms. J Neurosurg; 114(4):1154–1158

[39] Liu JK, Kan P, Karwande SV, Couldwell WT. Conduits for cerebrovascular bypass and lessons learned from the cardiovascular experience. Neurosurg Focus; 14(3):e3

[40] Bourassa MG, Fisher LD, Campeau L, Gillespie MJ, McConney M, Lespérance J. Long-term fate of bypass grafts: the Coronary Artery Surgery Study (CASS) and Montreal Heart Institute experiences. Circulation; 72(6 Pt 2):V71–V78

[41] Kim LJ, Tariq F, Sekhar LN. Pediatric bypasses for aneurysms and skull base tumors: short- and long-term outcomes. J Neurosurg Pediatr; 11(5):533–542

[42] Jung JM, Oh CW, Song KS, Bang JS. Emergency in situ bypass during middle cerebral artery aneurysm surgery: middle cerebral artery-superficial temporal artery interposition graft-middle cerebral artery anastomosis. J Korean Neurosurg Soc; 51(5):292–295

[43] Park ES, Ahn JS, Park JC, Kwon DH, Kwun BD, Kim CJ. STA-ACA bypass using the contralateral STA as an interposition graft for the treatment of complex ACA aneurysms: report of two cases and a review of the literature. Acta Neurochir (Wien); 154(8):1447–1453

[44] Kurobe H, Maxfield MW, Breuer CK, Shinoka T. Concise review: tissue-engineered vascular grafts for cardiac surgery: past, present, and future. Stem Cells Transl Med; 1(7):566–571

[45] Campbell GR, Campbell JH. Development of tissue engineered vascular grafts. Curr Pharm Biotechnol; 8(1):43–50

[46] Couldwell WT, Liu JK, Amini A, Kan P. Submandibular-infratemporal interpositional carotid artery bypass for cranial base tumors and giant aneurysms. Neurosurgery; 59(4) Suppl 2:ONS353–ONS359, discussion ONS359–ONS360

[47] Abla AA, Lawton MT. Anterior cerebral artery bypass for complex aneurysms: an experience with intracranial-intracranial reconstruction and review of bypass options. J Neurosurg; 120(6):1364–1377

[48] Tripathi P, Tripathi V, Naik RJ, Patel JM. Moya Moya cases treated with encephaloduroarteriosynangiosis. Indian Pediatr; 44(2):123–127

[49] Houkin K, Kuroda S, Ishikawa T, Abe H. Neovascularization (angiogenesis) after revascularization in moyamoya disease. Which technique is most useful for moyamoya disease? Acta Neurochir (Wien); 142(3):269–276

[50] Kinugasa K, Mandai S, Tokunaga K, et al. Ribbon enchephalo-duro-arteriomyo-synangiosis for moyamoya disease. Surg Neurol; 41(6):455–461

[51] Reis CV, Safavi-Abbasi S, Zabramski JM, Gusmão SN, Spetzler RF, Preul MC. The history of neurosurgical procedures for moyamoya disease. Neurosurg Focus; 20(6):E7

[52] Endo M, Kawano N, Miyaska Y, Yada K. Cranial burr hole for revascularization in moyamoya disease. J Neurosurg; 71(2):180–185

[53] Oliveira RS, Amato MC, Simão GN, et al. Effect of multiple cranial burr hole surgery on prevention of recurrent ischemic attacks in children with moyamoya disease. Neuropediatrics; 40(6):260–264

[54] Kalani MY, Elhadi AM, Ramey W, et al. Revascularization and pediatric aneurysm surgery. J Neurosurg Pediatr; 13(6):641–646

[55] Isono M, Ishii K, Kamida T, Inoue R, Fujiki M, Kobayashi H. Long-term outcomes of pediatric moyamoya disease treated by encephalo-duro-arterio-synangiosis. Pediatr Neurosurg; 36(1):14–21

[56] Yamada I, Matsushima Y, Suzuki S. Childhood moyamoya disease before and after encephalo-duro-arterio-synangiosis: an angiographic study. Neuroradiology; 34(4):318–322

[57] Adelson PD, Scott RM. Pial synangiosis for moyamoya syndrome in children. Pediatr Neurosurg; 23(1):26–33

[58] Suzuki R, Matsushima Y, Takada Y, Nariai T, Wakabayashi S, Tone O. Changes in cerebral hemodynamics following encephalo-duro-arterio-synangiosis (EDAS) in young patients with moyamoya disease. Surg Neurol; 31(5):343–349

[59] Golby AJ, Marks MP, Thompson RC, Steinberg GK. Direct and combined revascularization in pediatric moyamoya disease. Neurosurgery; 45(1):50–58, discussion 58–60

[60] Caldarelli M, Di Rocco C, Gaglini P. Surgical treatment of moyamoya disease in pediatric age. J Neurosurg Sci; 45(2):83–91

[61] Handa H, Yonekawa Y. Analysis of filing data bank of 1500 cases of spontaneous occlusion of the circle of Willis and follow-up study of 200 cases for more than 5 years. Stroke (Tokyo); 7:477–480

[62] Teo MK, Madhugiri VS, Steinberg GK. Editorial: Direct versus indirect bypass for moyamoya disease: ongoing controversy. J Neurosurg; 126(5):1520–1522

[63] Deng X, Gao F, Zhang D, et al. Direct versus indirect bypasses for adult ischemic-type moyamoya disease: a propensity score-matched analysis. J Neurosurg; 128(6):1785–1791

[64] Kim H, Jang DK, Han YM, et al. Direct bypass versus indirect bypass in adult moyamoya angiopathy with symptoms or hemodynamic instability: a meta-analysis of comparative studies. World Neurosurg; 94:273–284

[65] Kikuta K, Takagi Y, Fushimi Y, et al. "Target bypass": a method for preoperative targeting of a recipient artery in superficial temporal artery-to-middle cerebral artery anastomoses. Neurosurgery; 62(6) Suppl 3:1434–1441

[66] Wanebo JE, Zabramski JM, Spetzler RF. Superficial temporal artery-to-middle cerebral artery bypass grafting for cerebral revascularization. Neurosurgery; 55(2):395–398, discussion 398–399

[67] Yoshimura S, Egashira Y, Enomoto Y, Yamada K, Yano H, Iwama T. Superficial temporal artery to middle cerebral artery double bypass via a small craniotomy: technical note. Neurol Med Chir (Tokyo); 50(10):956–959

[68] Chater N, Spetzler R, Tonnemacher K, Wilson CB. Microvascular bypass surgery. Part 1: anatomical studies. J Neurosurg; 44(6):712–714

[69] Ikezaki K, Loftus CM, eds. Moyamoya Disease. Rolling Meadows, IL: American Association of Neurological Surgeons; 2001

[70] Connolly ES, McKhann GM II, Komotar RJ, Mocco J, Choudhri AF. Fundamentals of operative techniques in neurosurgery. New York, NY: Thieme; 2010

[71] Takagi Y, Kikuta K, Nishimura M, Ishii A, Nozaki K, Hashimoto N. Early experience of indocyanine green videoangiography in cerebrovascular surgery. Surg Cerebr Stroke.; 37(2):104–108

[72] Miyamoto S, Kikuchi H, Karasawa J, Nagata I, Ikota T, Takeuchi S. Study of the posterior circulation in moyamoya disease. Clinical and neuroradiological evaluation. J Neurosurg; 61(6):1032–1037

[73] Jin SC, Kwon DH, Song Y, Kim HJ, Ahn JS, Kwun BD. Multimodal treatment for complex intracranial aneurysms: clinical research. J Korean Neurosurg Soc; 44(5):314–319

[74] Ikeda A, Yamamoto I, Sato O, Morota N, Tsuji T, Seguchi T. Revascularization of the calcarine artery in moyamoya disease: OA-cortical PCA anastomosis—case report. Neurol Med Chir (Tokyo); 31(10):658–661

[75] Touho H, Karasawa J, Ohnishi H, Kobitsu K. Anastomosis of occipital artery to posterior cerebral artery with interposition of superficial temporal artery using occipital interhemispheric transtentorial approach: case report. Surg Neurol; 44(3):245–249, discussion 249–250

[76] Chang SW, Abla AA, Kakarla UK, et al. Treatment of distal posterior cerebral artery aneurysms: a critical appraisal of the occipital artery-to-posterior cerebral artery bypass. Neurosurgery; 67(1):16–25, discussion 25–26

[77] Pisapia JM, Walcott BP, Nahed BV, Kahle KT, Ogilvy CS. Cerebral revascularization for the treatment of complex intracranial aneurysms of the posterior circulation: microsurgical anatomy, techniques and outcomes. J Neurointerv Surg; 3(3):249–254

[78] Fukuda H, Evins AI, Burrell JC, Stieg PE, Bernardo A. A safe and effective technique for harvesting the occipital artery for posterior fossa bypass surgery: a cadaveric study. World Neurosurg; 82(3–4):e459–e465

[79] Martin NA. The use of extracranial-intracranial bypass for the treatment of giant and fusiform aneurysms. J Stroke Cerebrovasc Dis; 6(4):242–245

[80] Greene KA, Anson JA, Spetzler RF. Giant serpentine middle cerebral artery aneurysm treated by extracranial-intracranial bypass. Case report. J Neurosurg; 78(6):974–978

[81] Sekhar LN, Bucur SD, Bank WO, Wright DC. Venous and arterial bypass grafts for difficult tumors, aneurysms, and occlusive vascular lesions: evolution of surgical treatment and improved graft results. Neurosurgery; 44(6):1207–1223, discussion 1223–1224

[82] Gonzalez LF, Patterson DL, Lekovic GP, Nakaji P, Spetzler RF. Endoscopic harvesting of the radial artery for neurovascular bypass. Neurosurg Focus; 24(2):E10

[83] Hendrikse J, van der Zwan A, Ramos LM, Tulleken CA, van der Grond J. Hemodynamic compensation via an excimer laser-assisted, high-flow bypass before and after therapeutic occlusion of the internal carotid artery. Neurosurgery; 53(4):858–863, discussion 863–865

[84] Patel HC, Teo M, Higgins N, Kirkpatrick PJ. High flow extra-cranial to intracranial bypass for complex internal carotid aneurysms. Br J Neurosurg; 24(2):173–178

11 Case Examples of Cerebrovascular Bypass

M. Yashar S. Kalani, Ken-ichiro Kikuta, and Evgenii Belykh

Abstract

This chapter illustrates typically encountered clinical scenarios in which direct bypass procedures are indicated and presents clinical rationale for the choice of bypass procedure.

Keywords: atherosclerotic vascular occlusive disease, bypass, cerebral aneurysm, extracranial-intracranial, indications, moyamoya disease, skull base tumors

11.1 Bypass Indication for Atherosclerotic Occlusive Diseases

Atherosclerosis is a common disease that leads to the progressive stenosis and occlusion of cerebral vessels. Patients with transient ischemic attacks (TIAs) and cerebral infarctions due to the atherosclerotic stenosis of the internal carotid artery (ICA) and its branches usually present with general atherosclerosis. Studies on the natural history of ICA stenosis indicate that the annual stroke rate after diagnosis may vary from 3 to 27% per year.[1] Extracranial-intracranial (EC-IC) bypass aims to revascularize the affected hemisphere. New approaches for measuring brain blood flow and metabolism facilitate the selection of candidates in whom bypass surgery would probably improve outcome. Measurements of cerebral blood flow (CBF) and cerebrovascular resistance (CVR) by single-photon emission computed tomography (SPECT) (▶ Fig. 11.1) were unified using stereotactic brain coordinates and three-dimensional stereotactic surface projections by Mizumura et al.[2]

Hemodynamic compromise of ipsilateral artery occlusion is divided into three stages (stages 0–2)[3] based on CVR calculated from the CBF values at rest and during Diamox challenge (▶ Table 11.1).

Stage 2, or *misery perfusion*,[4] is considered to serve as criteria for the indication for revascularization. In symptomatic major cerebral artery disease, misery perfusion remains a predictor of subsequent stroke.[5] However, certain quantitative determinations of misery perfusion by different approaches (e.g., arterial spin labeling, magnetic resonance imaging [MRI], SPECT, and positron emission tomography [PET]) are still being debated. Patients with atherosclerotic occlusion of main brain arteries who satisfy the following eligibility categories can be candidates for bypass surgery according to the Carotid Occlusion Surgery Study[6] and the Japanese EC-IC Bypass Trial (JET)[7]:

1. Symptomatic ICA occlusion
2. Symptomatic middle cerebral artery (MCA) occlusion or severe stenosis
3. Age less than 73 years
4. Rankin disability scale 1 or 2
5. CBF less than 80% and CVR less than 10% (▶ Fig. 11.1) (or PET criteria: contralateral oxygen extraction fraction [OEF] ratio in the MCA territory > 1.130)
6. Angiographic confirmation of the ICA occlusion and presence of suitable intra- and extracranial vessels for anastomosis

Nevertheless, superficial temporal artery (STA) to MCA bypass plus best medical care failed to show more benefit than best medical care alone for the treatment of symptomatic intracranial occlusion in the JET[7] and the Carotid Occlusion Surgery Study.[6] The results of these studies have been interpreted by some authors as the end of the role for EC-IC bypass in the management of stroke. Although a general expansion of EC-IC bypass application in this population would not be supported by the results of trials, a selective subset of patients with medically refractory hemodynamic symptoms may obtain benefit from surgery with sufficiently low perioperative morbidity.[8]

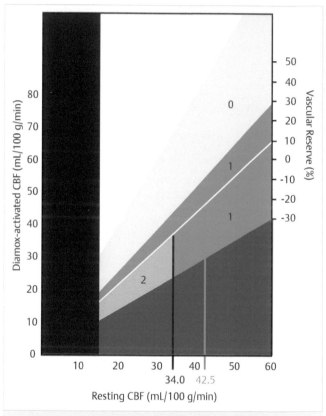

Fig. 11.1 Scale for assessment of resting cerebral blood flow (CBF) (x-axis) and Diamox-activated CBF (left y-axis). The Japanese EC-IC Bypass Trial indicated normal resting CBF as 42.5 mL/100 g/min (*vertical light blue line*). Resting CBF of < 80% is < 34.0 mL/100 g/min (*vertical purple line*). Quantitative value of vascular reserve is pointed from the left y-axis. The oblique line from this point to the right y-axis shows the rate of CBF increase after Diamox challenge. Stage 2 (*orange*) defines the area with < 80% resting CBF and < 10% vascular reserve. In such cases, surgery is indicated. In stage 1 (*light blue*), blood flow is impaired, but surgery is not more beneficial than conservative treatment. In stage 0 (*yellow*), there is normal autoregulation, and there are no indications for surgery. Purple and dark blue areas designate nonexistent combinations of resting CBF and Diamox-activated CBF. (Reproduced with permission from Tsuda K, Shiiya N, Washiyama N, et al. Carotid stenosis with impaired brain flow reserve is associated with an increased risk of stroke in on-pump cardiovascular surgery. Interact Cardiovasc Thorac Surg. 2018;27:75–80.)

Table 11.1 Classification of brain hemodynamic compromise

Stage	Hemodynamic compromise of ipsilateral artery occlusion[a]	Brain ischemia classification by SPECT[b]
0	Normal cerebral hemodynamics	Resting CBF ≥ 15 mL/100 g/min and CVR ≥ 30%
1	Autoregulatory vasodilation	34 mL/100 g/min (80% of normal CBF) > resting CBF ≥ 15 mL/100 g/min and 30% > CVR ≥ 10% or Resting CBF ≥ 34 mL/100 g/min and 30% > CVR ≥ –30%
2	Autoregulatory failure (increased OEF), also termed *misery perfusion*	34 mL/100 g/min > resting CBF ≥ 15 mL/100 g/min and 10% > CVR ≥ –30%

[a]Criteria from Powers et al.[3]
[b]Data from Mizumura et al.[2]
Abbreviations: CBF, cerebral blood flow; CVR, cerebrovascular reserve; OEF, oxygen extraction fraction; SPECT, single-photon emission computed tomography.

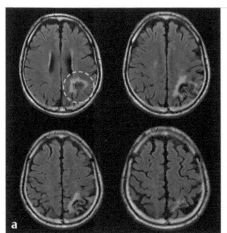
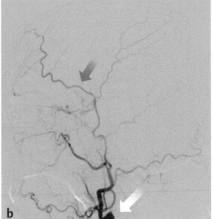
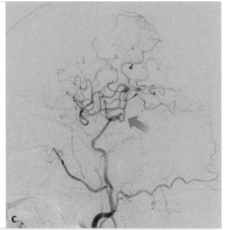

Fig. 11.2 Case 1. **(a)** FLAIR magnetic resonance image showing old ischemic lesion in the left parietal lobe (*dashed circle*). **(b)** Preoperative lateral digital subtractive left common carotid (CC) arteriogram showing stump of occluded internal carotid artery (*white arrow*) and donor superficial temporal artery branch (*blue arrow*). **(c)** Postoperative lateral digital subtractive left CC arteriogram showing the site of anastomosis (*blue arrow*) and rich blood flow through the middle cerebral artery branches. (Used with permission from University of Fukui, Japan.)

11.2 Illustrative Case 1: Atherosclerotic Internal Carotid Artery Occlusion

11.2.1 History

This 55-year-old man had unstable angina pectoris and underwent stenting of the coronary artery in June 2010. During the procedure, a left ICA occlusion was found. The patient was neurologically intact. During the follow-up examination 11 months later, restenosis of the coronary artery was revealed, and coronary artery off-pump bypass was indicated. But because off-pump bypass is associated with a risk of brain infarction due to ICA occlusion, the patient proceeded to CBF examination.

11.2.2 Examination

MRI showed old ischemic changes in the left hemisphere (▶ Fig. 11.2). PET (O[15] gas) before surgery showed stage 1 vasodilatory changes in the left cerebral hemisphere (▶ Table 11.2).

11.2.3 Operation

In July 2011, a double STA-MCA bypass was performed with no postoperative neurological deficit. The technique for harvesting the STA and its anastomosis to an M4 branch has been described in Chapter 9.

11.2.4 Postoperative Course

Postoperative gas-PET examination revealed increase of CVR in the left MCA territory. Two months later, the patient successfully underwent an off-pump coronary artery bypass. He was neurologically intact and angina pectoris significantly decreased during the follow-up period of 1 year.

11.3 Indications of Bypass for Moyamoya Disease and Moyamoya Syndrome

Moyamoya is a unique cerebrovascular disease of progressive stenosis of the bilateral terminal ICAs with development of rich

Table 11.2 O^{15} gas and water PET brain examination in case 1

MCA cortical territory	Normal	Preoperative		Postoperative	
		Left	Right	Left	Right
CBF (mL/100 g/min)	>32	41.2	47.0	40.9	46.0
CMRO$_2$ (mL/100 g/min)	>2.3	2.98	3.10	2.75	2.77
OEF (%)	<52	50.6	46.1	55.2	49.3
CBV (mL/100 g)	...	4.86	4.09	4.99	4.27
CBF/CBV	...	8.77	12.1	8.65	11.1
Diamox-activated CBF (mL/100 g/min)	...	36.4	54.9	43.0	55.1
CVR (%)	>10.5	**−11.7**	16.8	**5.0**	19.7

Abbreviations: CBF, cerebral blood flow; CBV, cerebral blood volume; CMRO$_2$, cerebral metabolic rate of oxygen; CVR, cerebrovascular reserve; MCA, middle cerebral artery; OEF, oxygen extraction fraction; PET, positron emission tomography.
Note: Significant decrease in CVR was revealed on preoperative examination. Postoperative data showed increase of global OEF, probably due to anemia and improvement of CVR in left MCA territory. The abnormal left preoperative CVR value and the improved postoperative value are shown in bold for comparison.

arterial collaterals at the base of the brain. Moyamoya disease should be distinguished from moyamoya syndrome according to the diagnostic criteria.[9] Bypass surgery is indicated for both conditions.

Moyamoya disease is found mostly among Japanese and other Asian populations, with an annual prevalence of 6.03 to 10.5 cases per 100,000 individuals in Japan.[10] The distribution of the age of ischemic onset demonstrates two peaks, one at 5 to 9 years of age and a lower peak at 35 to 39 years of age, whereas distribution of the age of hemorrhagic onset demonstrates a peak at 25 to 50 years of age.[10] Moyamoya disease is clinically progressive in most cases with childhood onset and is also progressive in many adult-onset cases. The common clinical scenario is repeated TIAs, cerebral infarctions, and brain atrophy in children and intracerebral hemorrhages from abnormal dilated lenticulostriate arteries or microaneurysms of abnormal moyamoya vessels or saccular aneurysms in adults. The explanation for such clinical presentations can be obtained from Suzuki's six-stage angiographic system of moyamoya disease.[11] Moyamoya disease shows more rapid clinical and angiographic progression in children than in adults, so it should be treated as soon as possible. In pediatric patients, surgery is indicated even for the asymptomatic hemispheres because of a strong possibility that it will become symptomatic in the near future. In adults, however, close follow-up observation is recommended, because asymptomatic adults usually have a good prognosis without bypass.[12] From the clinical point of view, many cases with stenosis of the arteries that form the circle of Willis can be difficult to distinguish from cases of moyamoya disease, so the term moyamoya syndrome was introduced.[13]

Medical treatments have not been found to be effective in reversing the progression of arterial stenosis seen in moyamoya disease. Surgical treatment of moyamoya disease began in the mid-1970s when Yaşargil proposed anastomosis of the STA to a branch of the MCA.[14] EC-IC bypass can reverse the progression of ischemia when the ischemic state of the brain remains in a recoverable state. Surgical treatment is based on the clinical characteristics; anatomical findings on MRI, magnetic resonance angiography (MRA), computed tomography (CT), and angiography; and functional assessment of CBF with SPECT, PET, and acetazolamide challenge test. It is still controversial whether direct bypass is necessary for the treatment of moyamoya disease, because indirect revascularization is effective. Indeed, direct bypass between a small STA and a small MCA, especially in children, is not always easy and carries risk of perioperative complications. However, direct bypass is more reliable in reducing hemodynamic stress to the moyamoya vessels, and it is an indispensable procedure for adult patients. In fact, some authors reported no significant reduction of the rebleeding rate after bypass surgery,[15] so surgical treatment in adult hemorrhagic patients remains controversial. In rare cases with pronounced ischemia in anterior cerebral artery (ACA) territory, direct STA-ACA anastomosis is essential.

The treatment guidelines, published in 2009[16] and 2012,[17] stated the effectiveness of direct bypass for both pediatric and adult cases. Optimal treatment of moyamoya disease is now widely accepted to require collateral formation in both the MCA and either ACA or posterior cerebral artery (PCA) territories. Multiple treatment choices that include combined direct and indirect bypass surgery are applied for most pediatric cases of moyamoya disease.[18]

During the first month after bypass, approximately 30% of patients exhibit TIA. However, symptoms usually improve thereafter.[19,20]

11.4 Illustrative Case 2: Moyamoya Disease

11.4.1 History

A 30-year-old female patient with Down syndrome presented with a new onset of left-sided weakness.

11.4.2 Examination

On examination, the patient had mild weakness of the left arm and leg (4/5 on the Medical Research Council Scale for Muscle Strength). Imaging revealed evidence of right cerebral vascular accidents, severe hypoperfusion of the right cerebral hemisphere, and stenosis of the right internal carotid artery consistent with moyamoya disease (▶ Fig. 11.3).[21]

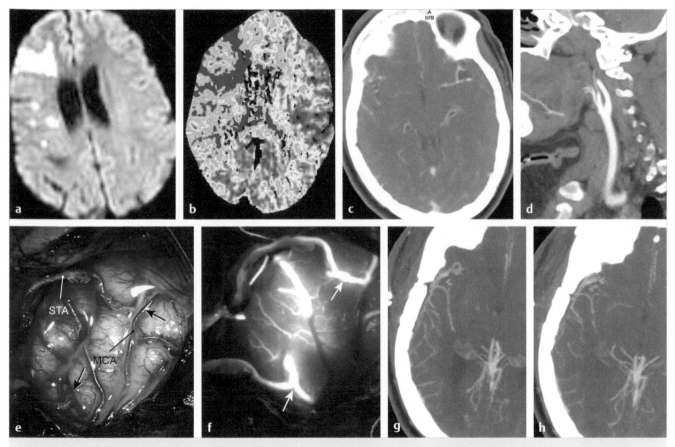

Fig. 11.3 Case 2, illustrating bypass for treatment of moyamoya disease. A 30-year-old female patient with Down syndrome presented with a new onset of left-sided weakness. **(a)** Diffusion-weighted axial magnetic resonance image demonstrates evidence of prior right cerebral vascular accidents. **(b)** Computed tomography (CT) perfusion depicts severe hypoperfusion of the right cerebral hemisphere, while CT angiograms of the **(c)** head and **(d)** neck demonstrate severe intracranial right internal carotid artery stenosis. The patient received a diagnosis of moyamoya disease. A right superficial temporal artery (STA) to middle cerebral artery (MCA) bypass was performed to revascularize the intracranial circulation. **(e)** Intraoperative image demonstrates a double-barrel STA-MCA bypass (*arrows*). **(f)** Indocyanine green angiography demonstrates patency of the bypasses. **(g, h)** CT angiograms of the head demonstrate patency of the bypass. The patient awoke at neurological baseline.

11.4.3 Operation

The patient underwent STA-MCA double bypass. The operative technique was the same as that described in Chapter 10, Section 10.3.1.

11.4.4 Postoperative Course

The patient awoke at neurological baseline. At the 1-month follow-up, the patient had slightly improved left-sided weakness (4 + /5).

11.5 Indications for Bypass in Complex and Giant Aneurysms

Arterial intracranial aneurysms are lesions with potentially devastating consequences. The goal of treating any aneurysm is to prevent bleeding by exclusion of the aneurysm from circulation. The most common treatment strategies for intracranial arterial aneurysms include endovascular occlusion and micro-surgical clipping. Both treatments have their pros and cons. In certain situations, such as giant blister-like[22] or dissecting aneurysms, proximal occlusion or trapping of the parent artery is required. If a dramatic decrease in blood flow after trapping is suspected, or if the balloon test occlusion documents that the patient may not tolerate permanent parent artery occlusion, bypass surgery should be considered prior to trapping to prevent ischemia. Patients with such complicated aneurysms who need vascular reconstruction are rare.[23,24,25,26] Attempts of bypass application for treatment of difficult cerebral aneurysms have increased since Yaşargil introduced microvascular techniques in neurosurgery, but the first "high-flow" bypass was performed without a microscope and was reported by Lougheed et al[27,28] in 1971. Sato and Kadoya[29] mentioned application of saphenous vein grafts beginning in 1974 for occlusive disease, traumatic occlusion of the ICA, and intracranial aneurysms. In 1979, Iwabuchi et al[30] reported a case of a giant ICA aneurysm treated with a long-vein bypass graft and trapping of the ICA. Many different techniques and nuances in high-flow bypass exist throughout the neurosurgical centers in the world. In recent published articles on EC-IC bypass application for the treatment of patients with complex intracranial aneurysms, good graft patency rates were achieved with low surgical morbidity and mortality.[23,31]

11.6 Illustrative Case 3: Giant Arterial Aneurysm

11.6.1 History

A 7-year-old boy presented with headache and lethargy. His medical history was unremarkable, and he was otherwise healthy (▶ Fig. 11.4).

11.6.2 Examination

The patient was neurologically intact. MRI demonstrated a giant dissecting posterior cerebral artery aneurysm. A balloon test occlusion failed, and the patient was scheduled for bypass to the distal PCA and sacrifice of the parent vessel.

11.6.3 Operation

The patient underwent STA to distal PCA bypass using an orbitozygomatic craniotomy. This bypass was followed by occlusion of the PCA immediately beyond the fusiform segment of the vessel.

11.6.4 Postoperative Course

Postoperative imaging revealed a significant reduction in the size of the aneurysm. The patient had a difficult postoperative course but ultimately recovered completely.

11.7 Indications for Bypass Skull Base Tumors

Because of improvements in chemoradiotherapy regimens, the indications for performing bypass for skull base tumors have greatly decreased.[21] Specifically, for malignant anterior and

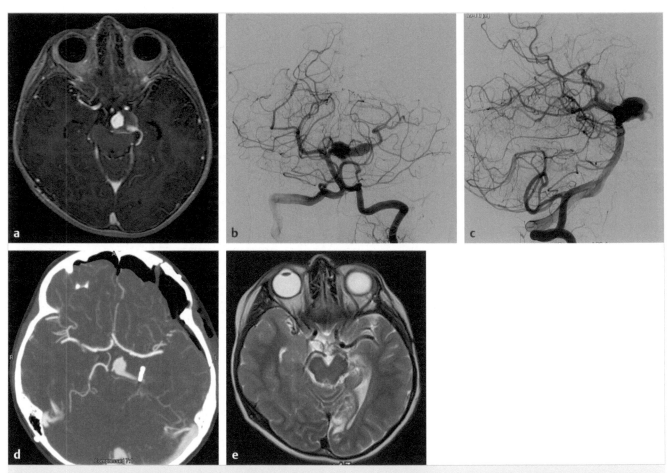

Fig. 11.4 Case 3, illustrating bypass for treatment of complex cerebral aneurysms. A 7-year-old boy presented with headache and lethargy. He was the result of a normal pregnancy and was otherwise healthy. Axial T2-weighted magnetic resonance imaging (MRI) (a), anteroposterior angiogram (b), and lateral vertebral artery angiogram (c) reveal a fusiform giant posterior cerebral artery (PCA) aneurysm with mass effect upon the brainstem. The patient underwent a superficial temporal artery to PCA bypass distal to the fusiform segment of the vessel followed by distal vessel sacrifice. (d) Postoperative axial computed tomographic angiography demonstrates significant reduction in the mass of the aneurysm. Postoperatively, the patient had a cerebrovascular accident from which he made a complete recovery. (e) One-year follow-up axial T1-weighted MRI reveals resolution of the mass effect.

middle fossa pathology, chemoradiotherapy affords survival benefits similar to those associated with aggressive resection of the tumor, skull base, and ICA (followed by revascularization).[32] Nonetheless, there remain select cases of skull base pathology, usually benign tumors such as meningiomas and chondrosarcomas, where vessel involvement by tumor may necessitate sacrifice of the intracranial circulation.[33] In cases where vessel sacrifice has to be performed proximally, a high-flow bypass is necessary to revascularize the distal circulation to prevent ischemia. In these cases, the choice of bypass is often an external carotid artery (ECA) to MCA bypass using a radial artery or saphenous vein graft. More recently, we have begun using an internal maxillary artery to MCA bypass using a radial artery graft. Although this graft provides less flow, the shorter length of the bypass ensures a higher rate of patency.

11.8 Illustrative Case 4: Bypass in the Setting of Skull Base Tumor

11.8.1 History

A 48-year-old man presented with a history of clival chondrosarcoma (▶ Fig. 11.5a–c). The lesion was treated in 2002 at an outside institution with Gamma Knife (Elekta AB) radiosurgery. The lesion had initially responded well to radiosurgery in 2005 (▶ Fig. 11.5d–e) but demonstrated increased growth on follow-up MRI in 2007 and subsequently in 2011 (▶ Fig. 11.5f–g). In 2011, the patient underwent an endoscopic transnasal approach for debulking of the tumor (▶ Fig. 11.5h–j). In 2013, follow-up MRI (not shown) revealed regrowth of the tumor, which was treated with additional Gamma Knife radiosurgery. In 2014, the patient developed TIAs.

11.8.2 Examination

The patient was neurologically intact but experienced episodic TIAs. MRI revealed compression of the right ICA by tumor (▶ Fig. 11.5k–m); this was confirmed on formal angiography.

11.8.3 Operation

The patient underwent a right mini-orbitozygomatic craniotomy for a high-flow, ECA-MCA bypass using a radial artery graft (▶ Fig. 11.5n, o).

11.8.4 Postoperative Course

Postoperative angiography (▶ Fig. 11.5p–r) demonstrated patency of the bypass. The patient had resolution of the TIAs.

11.9 Discussion

The first three illustrative cases demonstrate the use of low-flow bypass for treatment of various pathologies. For atherosclerotic patients, the craniotomy should be as small as is needed because minimal invasiveness is beneficial in elderly patients. High-flow bypass has no role in the treatment of cerebral ischemia because only a slight increase in blood flow to preexisting collaterals is needed, and high-flow bypass may be dangerous in a chronic ischemic brain because of the risk of hyperperfusion or hemorrhage.

In case 1, the patient presented with TIAs due to right MCA stenosis. Here the patient was medically refractory and required bypass to treat cerebral ischemia. Double bypass was chosen in this case because of severe MCA stenosis. We could increase blood flow in both supra- and infrasylvian portions of the MCA using two separate grafts. After surgery, the patient exhibited TIAs, which are common complications in the postoperative course of bypass surgery.

In case 2, the utility of bypass procedures in patients with moyamoya is demonstrated. When possible, we prefer to perform both direct and indirect revascularization of patients with moyamoya to optimize their likelihood of recovery and improvement.

Measuring of CBF and metabolism is essential for the identification of the appropriate surgical revascularization procedure. SPECT scans with acetazolamide are thought to be the most sensitive approach in the evaluation of CBF functional reserve in the JET study.[2] Gas-PET (O_2 extraction) gives information about brain tissue demand and is also a tool of assessment.[34,35] Another new method of CBF assessment using MRI is arterial spin labeling, which magnetically labels flowing spins in the proximal arteries.[36] Arterial spin labeling does not require radioactive medications, but its specificity and accuracy for measurement of brain blood flow and metabolism require further study. In the four cases presented in this chapter, CBF was measured with gas-PET. Sensitivity and specificity of arterial spin labeling for CBF measurement after bypass surgery have not yet been defined. In case 1, arterial spin labeling investigation had not revealed blood flow changes (*images are not shown*), but PET showed an increase of CVR.

Local CBF usually increases after bypass surgery. During the first month after bypass, approximately 30% of patients experience TIAs, which are probably attributable to the insufficiency of autoregulation of intracranial arterial flow. A syndrome of cerebral hyperperfusion occurs after the operation in approximately 30% of patients with moyamoya disease and in fewer patients with atherosclerotic vascular occlusive diseases. Hyperperfusion is determined as quantitative two times increase of CBF compared with CBF before surgery and can cause severe complications, such as brain edema and hemorrhage.[37] Due to the anatomy of donor and recipient arteries, high-flow bypasses cause deterioration of cerebral hyperperfusion more frequently than low-flow bypasses. Therefore, postoperative blood-flow measurement and specialized medical treatment are mandatory to prevent both ischemic and hyperperfusion complications.[38,39]

Case 3 illustrates the bypass techniques available in the treatment strategy for aneurysms. In this case, a balloon test occlusion failed. Given the results of the balloon test occlusion and the young age of the patient, he was considered for revascularization and parent vessel sacrifice. The patient underwent an STA to distal PCA bypass to revascularize the distal PCA territory followed by occlusion of the PCA distal to the aneurysm. In the absence of flow, this strategy results in thrombosis of the aneurysm with excellent outcomes and low morbidity.[23,31] The brain blood flow demands should be carefully studied when choosing an adequate bypass technique.

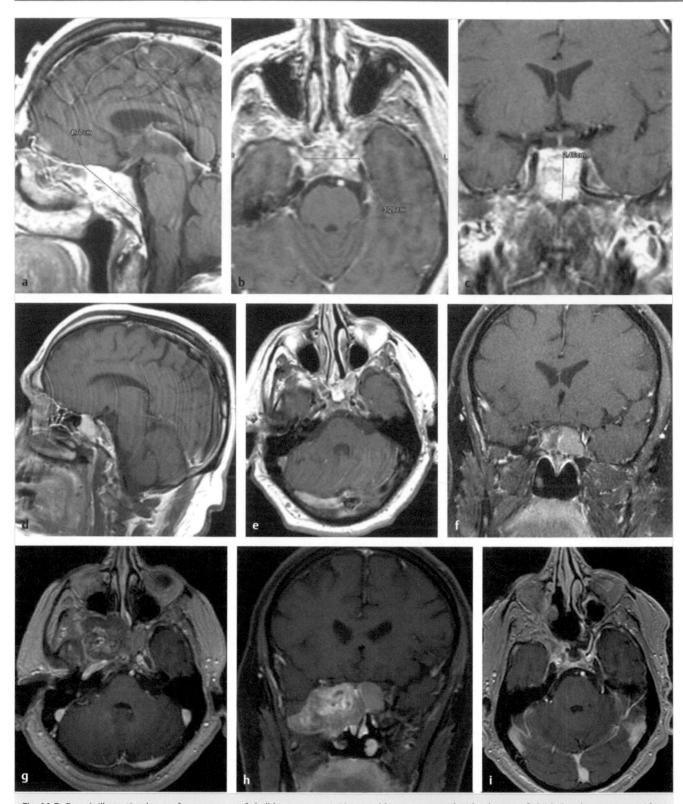

Fig. 11.5 Case 4, illustrating bypass for treatment of skull base tumor. A 48-year-old man presented with a history of clival chondrosarcoma, evident on **(a)** sagittal, **(b)** axial, and **(c)** coronal postcontrast magnetic resonance imaging (MRI). The patient had an initial favorable response to radiosurgery, as indicated by postcontrast MRI **(d, e)** showing a decrease in tumor size. However, the tumor demonstrated increased growth on follow-up **(f)** coronal and **(g)** axial MRI. Further growth ultimately necessitated an endoscopic debulking of the tumor as shown in **(h)** preoperative coronal, **(i)** postoperative axial, and (*continued*)

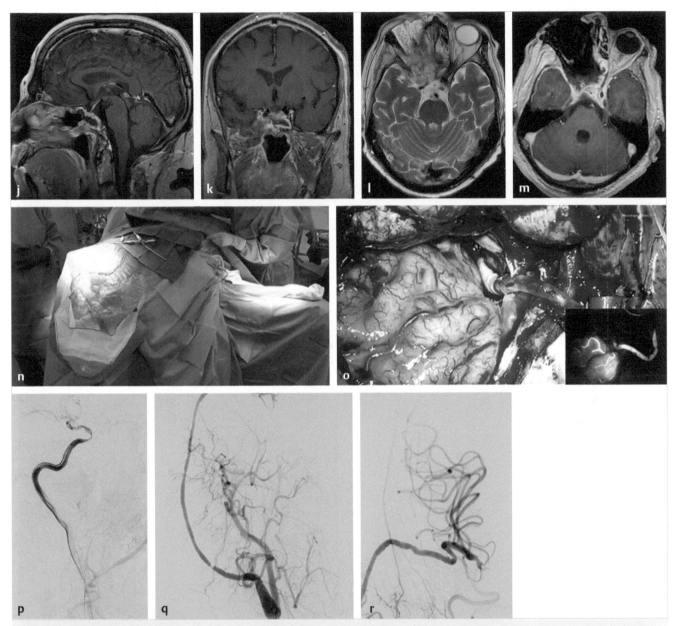

Fig. 11.5 (*continued*) (**j**) sagittal MRIs. After this resection, the patient continued to do well but gradually began complaining of episodic transient ischemic attacks (TIAs). MRI revealed compression of the right internal carotid artery by tumor (**k–m**) confirmed on formal angiography. The patient underwent a right-sided mini-orbitozygomatic craniotomy for external carotid to middle cerebral artery bypass using a radial artery graft. (**n**) Intraoperative setup and patient positioning. (**o**) Intraoperative microscope view of the cranial approach after bypass completion, with inset indocyanine green angiogram. (**p–r**) Postoperative angiography revealed patency of the bypass, and the patient had resolution of his TIAs.

Indications for performing bypass for resection of aggressive skull base tumors are rapidly decreasing.[21] With improvements in chemoradiotherapy, these cases are likely to be treated using only these modalities. In select cases of benign skull base pathology, there remains a role for aggressive resection of the involved vessel, followed by revascularization. These endeavors often require the use of a high-flow bypass, because the intracranial circulation is often sacrificed proximally, as illustrated by case 4.

11.10 Conclusion

Bypass surgery is an elegant and useful skill set that is best mastered in the laboratory using graded practice. Despite advances in medical management, endovascular techniques, and chemoradiotherapy, bypass surgery remains an essential tool for treatment of select cases of cerebral ischemia, complex aneurysms not amenable to endovascular techniques, and skull base tumors with vascular involvement. Practitioners are urged to maintain bypass techniques in their armamentarium of training as these skills may become necessary in emergency situations where comfort with vascular reconstruction may be the difference between a good outcome and a poor outcome for the patient.

References

[1] Spetzler RF. Cerebral revascularization for stroke. New York: Thieme-Stratton; 1985

[2] Mizumura S, Nakagawara J, Takahashi M, et al. Three-dimensional display in staging hemodynamic brain ischemia for JET study: objective evaluation using SEE analysis and 3D-SSP display. Ann Nucl Med; 18(1):13–21

[3] Powers WJ, Press GA, Grubb RL , Jr, Gado M, Raichle ME. The effect of hemodynamically significant carotid artery disease on the hemodynamic status of the cerebral circulation. Ann Intern Med; 106(1):27–34

[4] Baron JC, Bousser MG, Rey A, Guillard A, Comar D, Castaigne P. Reversal of focal "misery-perfusion syndrome" by extra-intracranial arterial bypass in hemodynamic cerebral ischemia. A case study with 15O positron emission tomography. Stroke; 12(4):454–459

[5] Yamauchi H, Higashi T, Kagawa S, et al. Is misery perfusion still a predictor of stroke in symptomatic major cerebral artery disease? Brain; 135(Pt 8):2515–2526

[6] Powers WJ, Clarke WR, Grubb RL , Jr, Videen TO, Adams HP , Jr, Derdeyn CP, COSS Investigators. Extracranial-intracranial bypass surgery for stroke prevention in hemodynamic cerebral ischemia: the Carotid Occlusion Surgery Study randomized trial. JAMA; 306(18):1983–1992

[7] Ogasawara K, Ogawa A. [JET study (Japanese EC-IC Bypass Trial)]. Nihon rinsho. Nihon Rinsho; 64 Suppl 7:524–527

[8] Amin-Hanjani S, Barker FG , II, Charbel FT, Connolly ES , Jr, Morcos JJ, Thompson BG, Cerebrovascular Section of the American Association of Neurological Surgeons, Congress of Neurological Surgeons. Extracranial-intracranial bypass for stroke-is this the end of the line or a bump in the road? Neurosurgery; 71(3):557–561

[9] Takahashi JC, Miyamoto S. Moyamoya disease: recent progress and outlook. Neurol Med Chir (Tokyo); 50(9):824–832

[10] Hoshino H, Izawa Y, Suzuki N, Research Committee on Moyamoya Disease. Epidemiological features of moyamoya disease in Japan. Neurol Med Chir (Tokyo); 52(5):295–298

[11] Suzuki J, Takaku A. Cerebrovascular "moyamoya" disease. Disease showing abnormal net-like vessels in base of brain. Arch Neurol; 20(3):288–299

[12] Yang J, Hong JC, Oh CW, et al. Clinicoepidemiological features of asymptomatic moyamoya disease in adult patients. J Cerebrovasc Endovasc Neurosurg; 16(3):241–246

[13] Phi JH, Wang KC, Lee JY, Kim SK. Moyamoya syndrome: a window of moyamoya disease. J Korean Neurosurg Soc; 57(6):408–414

[14] Yaşargil MG. Experimental small vessel surgery in the dog including patching and grafting of cerebral vessels and formation of functioning extra-intracranial shunts. In: Donaghy RMP, Yaşargil MG, eds. Microvascular surgery. Stuttgart: George-Thieme; 1967:87–126

[15] Yoshida Y, Yoshimoto T, Shirane R, Sakurai Y. Clinical course, surgical management, and long-term outcome of moyamoya patients with rebleeding after an episode of intracerebral hemorrhage: an extensive follow-up study. Stroke; 30(11):2272–2276

[16] Research of Intractable Diseases of the Ministry of Health. Labour Welfare, Japan. Recommendations for the Management of Moyamoya Disease: A Statement from Research Committee on Spontaneous Occlusion of the Circle of Willis (Moyamoya Disease). Surgery for Cerebral Stroke; 37(5):321–337

[17] Research Committee on the Pathology and Treatment of Spontaneous Occlusion of the Circle of Willis, Health Labour Sciences Research Grant for Research on Measures for Infractable Diseases. Guidelines for diagnosis and treatment of moyamoya disease (spontaneous occlusion of the circle of Willis). Neurol Med Chir (Tokyo); 52(5):245–266

[18] Matsushima T, Inoue K, Kawashima M, Inoue T. History of the development of surgical treatments for moyamoya disease. Neurol Med Chir (Tokyo); 52(5):278–286

[19] Funaki T, Takahashi JC, Takagi Y, et al. Unstable moyamoya disease: clinical features and impact on perioperative ischemic complications. J Neurosurg; 122(2):400–407

[20] Starke RM, Komotar RJ, Hickman ZL, et al. Clinical features, surgical treatment, and long-term outcome in adult patients with moyamoya disease. Clinical article. J Neurosurg; 111(5):936–942

[21] Kalani MY, Rangel-Castilla L, Ramey W, et al. Indications and results of direct cerebral revascularization in the modern era. World Neurosurg; 83(3):345–350

[22] Ishikawa T, Mutoh T, Nakayama N, et al. Universal external carotid artery to proximal middle cerebral artery bypass with interposed radial artery graft prior to approaching ruptured blood blister-like aneurysm of the internal carotid artery. Neurol Med Chir (Tokyo); 49(11):553–558

[23] Kalani MY, Ramey W, Albuquerque FC, et al. Revascularization and aneurysm surgery: techniques, indications, and outcomes in the endovascular era. Neurosurgery; 74(5):482–497, discussion 497–498

[24] Kalani MY, Zabramski JM, Nakaji P, Spetzler RF. Bypass and flow reduction for complex basilar and vertebrobasilar junction aneurysms. Neurosurgery; 72(5):763–775, discussion 775–776

[25] Kalani MY, Zabramski JM, Hu YC, Spetzler RF. Extracranial-intracranial bypass and vessel occlusion for the treatment of unclippable giant middle cerebral artery aneurysms. Neurosurgery; 72(3):428–435, discussion 435–436

[26] Spetzler RF, Fukushima T, Martin N, Zabramski JM. Petrous carotid-to-intradural carotid saphenous vein graft for intracavernous giant aneurysm, tumor, and occlusive cerebrovascular disease. J Neurosurg; 73(4):496–501

[27] Lougheed WM, Marshall BM, Hunter M, Michel ER, Sandwith-Smyth H. Common carotid to intracranial internal carotid bypass venous graft. Technical note. J Neurosurg; 34(1):114–118

[28] Yaşargil MG. Operative anatomy. In: Yaşargil MG, ed. Microsurgical Anatomy of the Basal Cisterns and Vessels of the Brain, Diagnostic Studies, General Operative Techniques and Pathological Considerations of the Intracranial Aneurysms. Vol. 1. Stuttgart and New York: Verlag GT; 1984:72–134

[29] Sato S, Kadoya S. EC-IC bypass surgery using a long vein graft—reconstructive procedures for the occluded long vein grafts [in Japanese]. No Shinkei Geka; 15(8):885–890

[30] Iwabuchi T, Kudo T, Hatanaka M, Oda N, Maeda S. Vein graft bypass in treatment of giant aneurysm. Surg Neurol; 12(6):463–466

[31] Kalani MY, Elhadi AM, Ramey W, et al. Revascularization and pediatric aneurysm surgery. J Neurosurg Pediatr; 13(6):641–646

[32] Kalani MY, Kalb S, Martirosyan NL, et al. Cerebral revascularization and carotid artery resection at the skull base for treatment of advanced head and neck malignancies. J Neurosurg; 118(3):637–642

[33] Yang T, Tariq F, Chabot J, Madhok R, Sekhar LN. Cerebral revascularization for difficult skull base tumors: a contemporary series of 18 patients. World Neurosurg; 82(5):660–671

[34] Kikuta K. Experiences using 3-tesla magnetic resonance imaging in the treatment of moyamoya disease. Acta Neurochir Suppl (Wien); 103:123–126

[35] Kuroda S, Kashiwazaki D, Hirata K, Shiga T, Houkin K, Tamaki N. Effects of surgical revascularization on cerebral oxygen metabolism in patients with moyamoya disease: an 15O-gas positron emission tomographic study. Stroke; 45(9):2717–2721

[36] Tsujikawa T, Kimura H, Matsuda T, et al. Arterial transit time mapping obtained by pulsed continuous 3D ASL imaging with multiple post-label delay acquisitions: comparative study with PET-CBF in patients with chronic occlusive cerebrovascular disease. PLoS One; 11(6):e0156005

[37] Ogasawara K, Inoue T, Kobayashi M, et al. Cerebral hyperperfusion following carotid endarterectomy: diagnostic utility of intraoperative transcranial Doppler ultrasonography compared with single-photon emission computed tomography study. AJNR Am J Neuroradiol; 26(2):252–257

[38] Fujimura M, Niizuma K, Inoue T, et al. Minocycline prevents focal neurological deterioration due to cerebral hyperperfusion after extracranial-intracranial bypass for moyamoya disease. Neurosurgery; 74(2):163–170, discussion 170

[39] Fujimura M, Tominaga T. Significance of cerebral blood flow analysis in the acute stage after revascularization surgery for moyamoya disease. Neurol Med Chir (Tokyo); 55(10):775–781

12 Postscript

12.1

A neurosurgical operation is a duel between the neurosurgeon and the disease. As in the boxing ring, there are three basic ways to strike at your opponent. For the boxer, they are the jab, hook, and uppercut; for the neurosurgeon, they are dissection, hemostasis, and microsurgical suturing (▶ Fig. P.1).

The answer to the question of how to become a good neurosurgeon was given by Kikuchi et al.[1] and included three key points:

1. Basic microsurgical skills, such as dissection, hemostasis, and anastomosis, should be mastered on plastic tubes, cadaver vessels, and laboratory animals.
2. Good anatomical knowledge of different approaches should be obtained during cadaver dissection.
3. Manual skills should be consolidated when assisting with and performing surgery under the supervision of an experienced neurosurgeon-teacher.

Therefore, laboratory training plays an essential part in the formation of a neurosurgeon, because it allows one to achieve the first two goals. Microsurgical skills training and learning of surgical microanatomy are the personal responsibility of the trainee, whereas the tactics of patient treatment may be discussed with colleagues on rounds and at conferences.

We would like to end this monograph with a parable about calligraphy. Being a precise and delicate art, calligraphy, like neurosurgery, requires a long training curve. Watching a master neurosurgeon perform brain surgery is like watching the brushstrokes of a master of the art of calligraphy.

One young man wished to study calligraphy and went to a famous master to ask him to be his tutor. The calligrapher accepted him as his apprentice with great cordiality. After studying under the master for several years, the apprentice decided that there was no reason to stay with the master, because he had mastered the art of calligraphy well enough. He told the master about his intention to leave. The master did not try to persuade him to stay. Instead, he gave him a box and said at parting: I don t want anyone to have this box. Take it and bury it at the foot of the mountain. The young man took the box, said goodbye to the master, and left. The box was small but rather heavy. As he walked, the young man tried to guess what could be inside the box. Maybe there were treasures hidden inside? Finally, curiosity overpowered him. He unslung the box and put it on the ground. Fortunately, the box was sealed carelessly, and the young man opened the lid easily. He gaped in surprise, because the box held nothing but old inkwells! There were several dozen inkwells in the box. But the young man was most struck, not by the number of inkwells, but by the fact that there was a big hole worn through the bottom of each inkwell! That s how diligently his Master was working! The young man sat and looked through each inkwell for a long time. Then he quietly closed the lid, took the box on his shoulders, and resolutely went back to the reed hut of his master. From that time on, the apprentice devoted himself entirely to the art of calligraphy, without reservation. But it was only when his hair had turned completely gray that he achieved the peak and the true mastery came to him.[2]

How many inkwells have we worn through as neurosurgeons? It is no surprise that some of the techniques that we have been taught are not working well enough in our hands.

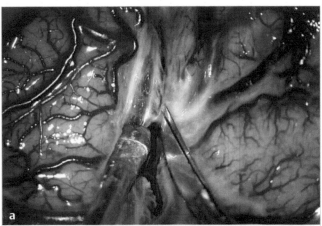

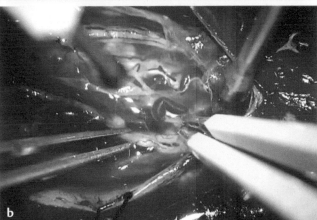

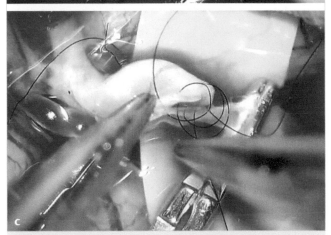

Fig. P.1 Three basic ways for the neurosurgeon to strike at the opponent. **(a)** Arachnoidal microdissection. **(b)** Hemostasis. **(c)** Microsurgical suturing.

There are numerous subtle nuances that we do not yet understand and which, when performed, make a difference. There are no miracles; only deliberate, persistent practice leads to the highest perfection. There is no best neurosurgeon and no best microneurosurgical technique. The way of perfection is endless.

Evgenii Belykh, MD
Phoenix, Arizona

References

[1] Kikuchi H. Illustrated Techniques in Microneurosurgery. Tokyo: Igaku-Shoin Medical Publisher; 1991

[2] Tarasov V. The Art of Management Control (in Your Pocket) [in Russian]. Moscow: Dobraya; 2009.

Index

Note: Page numbers set **bold** or *italic* indicate headings or figures, respectively.

A

anastomosis training
- arteriovenous fistula 76, 77
- deep operative field **76**, 77
- dry model **41**
- latex glove 42, *45*
- patency testing 65, *66*, **70**
- reconstruction, complex **77**, *78*, *109*
- skills assessment **91**
- synthetic microtubes **41**, *44–45*
- techniques 34–35
- types of anastamoses *44*, **47**
anesthesia, for animals **56**, 59, *59*
aneurysm clipping
- complications, errors **95**
- placenta model **83**, *84–86*
- skills assessment **91**
aneurysms, giant/complex case study **121**, *122*, **122**, 123
animal care
- anesthesia **56**, 59, *59*
- blood loss **56**, 60
- euthanasia **57**
- pain/distress symptoms **56**, 57, *58*
- principles **56**
- research, hazards in **58**
arterial spin labeling 123
aspirin dosages 94
atherosclerosis *118*, **118**, 119
atherosclertic ICA occlusion case study *119*, **119**, 120, 123

B

bayoneted microscissors
- defined 13, *15*
- dissection mastery **33**, *34–35*
- holding techniques *30*, **30**, *31–33*
beta-blockers 27
bipolar coagulation instruments **14**, *19*
bleeding errors **97**
blood flow replacement bypass **114**
blood-like solutions **87**
brain hemodynamic compromise classification 119
Brevital, anesthesia dosage regimen 59
bypass errors
- anesthesia-related issues **94**
- bleeding **97**
- craniotomy **95**
- donor vessel dissection **94**
- flow assessment **98**
- instruments **95**
- interrupted suture *97*, **97**
- knots/thread **96**
- operative field **95**
- OR environment/team **94**
- patient–treatment mismatch **94**
- postoperative period **98**
- recipient vessel selection **95**
- running sutures **96**
- types of **94**
- vessel grabbing **97**
- vessel preparation **95**, *96*
- wound closure **98**

C

cadaveric vessels **87**
carotid arteries approach *62*, **63**
carotid artery-interposition graft-MCA bypass **114**, *115*, **115**
Carotid Occlusion Surgery Study 94
carotid–jugular fistula, anastomosis technique **68**, *72*
case studies
- aneurysms, giant/complex **121**, *122*, **122**, 123
- atherosclerosis *118*, **118**, 119
- atherosclertic ICA occlusion *119*, **119**, 120, 123
- Moyamoya disease/syndrome **119**–**120**, *121*, **121**, 123
- skull base tumors **122**–**123**, *124–125*
cerebral hyperperfusion syndrome 123
chopsticks technique *28*, **28**, 33
clip appliers **14**, *18*, 24
clock principle *48*
combined bypass 104
constant hold, one suture exercise **37**, *39*
constant hold, same direction pulling exercise **37**, *40*
Coronary Artery Surgery Study 105
cottonoid *20*
counter-press method, suturing *46*, **46**
craniotomy **95**

D

deep operative field training
- anastomoses **76**, *77*
- dissection exercise **75**, *76*
- epineural suture *79*, **79**, *80*
- reconstruction, complex **77**, *78*, *109*
- simulation devices *22*, *23*, 75, *75*
- venous interposition graft/mismatched orifices **77**, *78*
Dexdomitor 59
Diprivan 59
donor vessel dissection errors **94**
donor vessel orifice shapes *51*
double-barrel bypass 104
drills, high-speed *22*, *23*
dry-laboratory training **87**
dyes *16*, *22*
dyes in patency testing 70

E

EC-IC bypass
- aim of *99*, **99**
- arterial basins, anastomosing *100*, **100**, *101–102*
- blood flow augmentation **107**
- blood flow volume *99*, *100*
- distal anastomosis options *104*, *109*
- distal anastomosis site *102*, *107*
- graft length *100*, *102–104*
- graft origin *105*, *110*
- graft pathway *105*, *110*
- indirect, general principles **105**, *111*
- laterality of **101**, *105–106*
- principles of *99*
- proximal anastomosis site *102*, *108*
- types of *99*
end-to-end anastomosis
- carotid/jugular, interrupted suture **68**, *72*
- double, arterial loop **68**, *71*
- principles *44–45*, *48–50*, **65**
- rat carotid exercise **47**, *67*, *70*
end-to-side anastomosis
- arteriovenous fistula 76, 77
- complications, errors 95
- continuous suture *66*, *68–69*
- principles **44**, *48*, *51*
exoscopes *10*, **10**
eyepiece diopter correction 7

F

field of clear view 8
fish-mouth technique *48*, *51*
flow assessment errors **98**
focal depth, of microscopes 8
focal distance 7
forceps
- described **11**, *12–13*, 24
- holding techniques *28*, *29*
- knot-tying exercises **11**, *13*
free groin flap/vascular pedicle *83*, **83**

G

Gas-PET 123

H

hemostasis *71*, *74*
human placenta **88**, *89*

I

index push technique
- forceps *28*, *29*
- long bayonet microscissors *32*
- scissors *29*, *30*
infection 95
instruments
- bayoneted 11, *17*, *19*, 24
- bayoneted microscissors 13, *15*
- bayoneted microscissors, holding techniques *30*, **30**, *31–33*
- bipolar coagulation **14**, *19*
- clip appliers **14**, *18*, 24
- complications, errors **95**
- costs of 24
- forceps **11**, *12–13*, 24
- forceps holding techniques *28*, *29*
- hand position *30*, *34*
- holding techniques *28*, **28**
- knot-tying forceps **11**, *13*
- long bayonet microscissors, holding techniques **30**
- maintenance of 11
- needle holders **11**, *12*
- overview **11**
- retractors **15**, *19*
- scalpels **14**, *18*
- scissors **13**, *14–16*
- scissors holding techniques *29*, *30*
- selection of 11
- skills assessment 91
- suction cannulas **15**, *20*
- tissue irrigators/solutions **15**
- training set 22, *24*
- vascular clips **13**, *17*
- vessel dilators *13*, **13**
- warm-up exercises **33**
interpupillary distance 6
interrupted suturing
- carotid/jugular, end-to-end anastomosis **68**, *72*
- complications, errors *97*, **97**
- running to interrupted *47*, **47**
- techniques **46**

J

Japanese EC-IC Bypass Trial 94

K

KEZLEX 42
kidney autotransplantation *81*, **81**, *82*
knot tying forceps **11**, *13*
knot tying on gauze
- constant hold, one suture **37**, *39*
- constant hold, same direction pulling **37**, *40*
- exercise 34, *36*, **36**, *37*
- skills assessment **91**
- snowflake exercise **38**, *42*
- suture end pushing **39**, *43*
- suture tails, simultaneous cutting **37**, *41*
- suture, intermittent grasping **36**, *38*
- suturing **36**
- untying knots **39**, *43*
knots/thread errors **96**

L

laboratory setup
- background material **16**
- costs of **22**, 24
- deep operative field simulation **22**, *23*
- drills, high-speed **22**, *23*
- dyes **16**, *22*
- materials/equipment **4**
- needles/sutures **16**, *20*, *21*, 24
- organization **4**, *5*
- purchasing alternatives **22**
- sponges/gauze **16**, *20*
LEGOs 75, *75*, 77
lift test 70
light intensity, of microscopes 8

M

magnification changer assembly 7
magnification, of microscopes 7, 9
MD-PVC Rat Model 42
microscopes
- costs of 24
- principles of operation *5*, **5**, *6–8*, 9, *9*

– setup **10**
– skills assessment 91
microsurgical training
– characteristics of good
  neurosurgeon 127
– extracurricular opportunities **90**
– hand position 27, *27*, **30**, *34*
– mental concentration **26**
– movement **1**, *2*
– muscle relaxation in 41
– operator position **26**
– post-clinical **90**
– practice schedule **89**
– preparation **2**, *6–7*, 8
– skill development stages **2**, *3*
– skills assessment 91, **91**
– structure of **90**
– surgical strategies 127, *127*
– techniques **26**
– terrain **1**
– tremor management 27, **27**
– warm-up exercises **33**
microvascular practice card 42, *44*
midline laparotomy training 63, **63**
milking test 70
misery perfusion 118
Moyamoya disease/syndrome 113,
  119–120, *121*, **121**, 123
muscle relaxation 41

N

needle bite assessment 91
needle handling/care assessment 91
needle holders **11**, *12*
needles/sutures **16**, 20, *21*, 24
Nembutal, anesthesia dosage
  regimen 59
nerve repair, epineural suture *79*, **79**,
  80

O

OA-PCA bypass **113**
occipital artery as donor vessel **114**
operative field issues **95**
operator positioning/posture
  assessment 91
optical parts, of microscopes *9*
OR environment/team errors **94**

P

patient–treatment mismatch **94**
pentothal, anesthesia dosage
  regimen 59
postoperative period errors **98**
poultry arteries **87**, *88*
pressurized models **87**
Promag 7
propranolol 27
pulsation test 70

R

R principles, animal care **56**
radial artery graft
– bypass skull tumors 122, *124–125*
– classification by origin 105
– complex reconstructions *109*
– distal anastomosis 104
– failures, causes of 105
– harvesting 114
– nomenclature 99
– proximal anastomosis 115
– STA-graft-A3-A4 bypass 113
Rapinovet, anesthesia dosage
  regimen 59
recipient vessel selection **95**
reconstruction, complex **77**, *78*, *109*
reduction principle 56
refinement principle 56
replacement principle 56
retractors **15**, *19*
reverse holding technique
– forceps 28, *29*
– long bayonet microscissors *31*
– scissors 29, *30*
robotic operative microscopes *5*, *7*
Rompun, anesthesia dosage
  regimen 59
running suturing
– complications, errors **96**
– running to interrupted *47*, **47**
– technique **47**, 50, *53–55*

S

saphenous vein graft
– aneurysms 121
– blood flow rates 100

– bypass skull tumors 122
– classification by origin 105
– failures, causes of 105
– nomenclature 99
– patency 100, 105
– proximal anastomosis 115
– selection of 114
– STA-graft-A3-A4 bypass 113
scalp necrosis 95
scalpels **14**, *18*
scissors **13**, *14–16*
scissors holding techniques **29**, *30*
side-to-side anastomosis
– femoral artery/vein, continuous
  suture **69**, *73*
– in situ reconstruction 100, *101–102*
– principles 44, **50**, *52–55*
skull base tumors **122–123**, *124–125*
snowflake exercise **38**, *42*
SPECT scans 123
STA-ACA bypass **113**
STA-MCA bypass **108**, **110**, *111*, **111**,
  112, **112**, *113*, **113**
STA-PCA bypass **113**
stereomicroscopes *5*, 8
suction cannulas **15**, *20*
supermicrosurgery *83*, **83**
surgical loupes **10**
sutures/needles **16**, 20, *21*, 24
suturing techniques
– anatomy 65
– complications, errors *66*, **96**, 97,
  97
– counter-press method *46*, **46**
– epineural suture *79*, **79**, *80*
– interrupted **46**
– knot-tying exercises **36**
– knots/thread errors **96**
– requirements 65
– running suturing **47**, *53–54*
– running suturing repair 50, *55*
– running to interrupted *47*, **47**
– skills assessment 91
– suture end pushing exercise **39**,
  43
– suture filaments sizes 20
– suture tails, simultaneous
  cutting **37**, *41*
synthetic microtubes, for anastomosis
  training **41**, *44*

T

Telazol, anesthesia dosage regimen
  59
tissue irrigators/solutions **15**
tissue respect assessment
  91
traction sutures, holding in place
  50
traditional technique
– forceps 28, *29*
– long bayonet microscissors *30*
– scissors 30, *30*

U

ultrasound in patency testing 70
untying knots **39**, *43*

V

Valium, anesthesia dosage regimen
  59
vascular clips **13**,
  17
Versed, anesthesia dosage regimen 59
vessel dilators *13*, **13**
vessel grabbing errors **97**
vessel handling assessment 91
vessel preparation errors **95**, *96*
video recording 8

W

warm-up exercises **33**
wet-laboratory training
– animal materials **89**
– cadaveric vessels **87**
– femoral neurovascular bundle
  approach *60*, **60**, *61*
– human placenta **88**, *89*
– midline laparotomy 63, **63**
– neck vessels approach *62*, **63**
– principles **58**
wound closure errors **98**

Z

zoom lens mechanism 7